STILL POSITIVE

a memoir

STILL POSITIVE

a memoir

JULIE LEWIS
WITH JENNY KOENIG

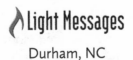
Light Messages

Durham, NC

Copyright © 2023 Julie Lewis and Jenny Koenig

Still Positive: a memoir
Julie Lewis with Jenny Koenig
https://stillpositive.com

Published 20232, by Torchflame Books
an Imprint of Light Messages Publishing
www.lightmessages.com
Durham, NC 27713 USA
SAN: 920-9298

Paperback ISBN: 978-1-61153-490-0
Hardcover ISBN: 978-1-61153-492-4
E-book ISBN: 978-1-61153-491-7
Library of Congress Control Number: 2023904230

This book is a memoir. It reflects the author's present recollections of experiences over a period of time. Some names and characteristics have been changed to protect the privacy of the people involved, some events have been compressed, and some dialogue has been recreated to capture the essence of the conversations to the best of the author's memory. All of the events in this story are factual and recalled and described to the best of the author's ability.

To the dream I dared to imagine;
Mylo, Rory, Fiona, Luna, Ramona and Ruby...
You are my miracle.

CONTENTS

INTRODUCTION

It's September 8, 2020. I am sitting in the kitchen watching my grandson's first-grade teacher trying to conduct his first day of online class for twenty-four six- and seven-year-olds. There is no manual. Online school has been thrust upon our world, an unwelcome gift of the COVID-19 pandemic.

This is a giant experiment, and the stakes are not low. So far, day one is a mini-disaster. But ... tomorrow will happen, and the day after that, online school is the new reality, indefinitely. Whether he likes it or not, Mr. Kratz and his fellow teachers will have to figure out how to promote learning this way because twenty-four kids, and their parents, are counting on him.

Online school is just a symptom of something much bigger, darker, and scarier. It's one of the everyday results of humanity trying to survive a global pandemic. Life with these fears and challenges is uncharted ground and daily life is a mixture of trying to find joy in the small things, like a baby's first step, while continually learning how to protect that baby from such a huge unknown threat.

As with COVID, what happens when you google your problem and there is no solution, no easy answer ... or no answer at all? Life without a manual, no guidebook available.

And what if that problem is huge, the most frightening challenge of your life? That's the world I was thrust into in 1990. Navigating the new diagnosis of AIDS with few answers, surrounded by fear, cloaked in stigma, and trying to survive day to day in unknown territory. It's a story of finding unlikely communities that helped me steer the way. **Living** in the moment while trying to be positive and authentic, and find real hope in the midst of daily uncertainty. **Learning** to let go of so many things, yet also learning to build a solid foundation for myself and my family, a foundation we could sink our feet into as life precariously shifted around us. **Leaning** into the love of God that never fails.

That is this book ... my life ... an imperfect science at best. And, for an ex-science teacher, the reality of so much trial and error ... oh, so much error ... is uncomfortable to say the least. But life is a great experiment and some of my greatest truth has come from my most difficult moments. This is an imperfect grace-filled journey of what has been my ungoogleable life.

PART 1

THERE WAS NO GUIDEBOOK

THE PHONE CALL

It's the end of the world as we know it and I feel fine

R.E.M.

Wednesday, August 15, 1990, was a normal summer morning, not a sunny day, but definitely summer, warm and muggy. Exhausted from packing our house into moving boxes, I sat on the front steps trying to catch my breath and muster up the energy to finish the task at hand. I stared at the flowers in the yard I was about to leave behind, gazing at our neighbors' houses and taking in the cul-de-sac that had been my world for the past four years. I thought my life was about to change drastically because we were moving to a new city, miles away. This seemed like a milestone, a big deal. I had no idea that in a few moments the definition of a "big deal" was going to be lifted to a different level. The direction of my life was about to take a major detour.

The phone rang in the kitchen.

When the conversation started with "You'd better sit down," I knew with certainty that it wasn't going to be good news.

I can still hear the voice of my doctor from Bellingham on the other end of the line. "Do you remember the blood transfusion you had when Teresa was born?"

"Yes," I replied.

"Well, this is probably nothing to worry about, because it

was six and a half years ago," he said, "but the blood bank just contacted me to inform us that one of the three people who donated blood for your blood transfusion now has AIDS."

I felt the blood draining out of my head as I stared at Scott from across our dining room table, making sure he could hear the whole conversation.

"They are suggesting that you get an HIV test."

Silence.

He went on, "Now, this donor could've been infected after your blood transfusion so don't get too worried about it yet. There's a good chance you're just fine."

Awkwardly ending the phone conversation, I looked at my husband for some hint of assurance that everything was going to be okay, that this was not real. He looked concerned, but in true Scott Lewis fashion, he hid any inclination to panic. Nonetheless, inwardly, in that same moment, I knew in my gut, absolutely, positively, that I was infected with HIV.

For more than a year, normal effort had made me unusually tired, exhausted really. I'd visited several doctors and each time they would look at me with calm, "parent-like" eyes and say, "Oh, you're just so busy. You have so much going on; you have three little kids. You're exhausting yourself; you need to get some rest."

But, deep down, I knew what being exhausted felt like. I chronically did "too much," always burning the candle at both ends. This was different. I started thinking about diseases the medical community didn't give much credibility to, like Chronic Fatigue Syndrome. I absolutely knew something was wrong with me, besides general tiredness.

His words went through my head again: "You should get an HIV test." This was the missing puzzle piece I had been searching for; this was what was wrong: I had HIV.

That call began the longest and hardest five days of my

life. Hanging up the phone, my entire perspective changed in a moment. Things that had been important an hour before meant nothing to me. I no longer cared if my dishes were packed securely or if the boxes were being stacked in the truck properly. I could sense my body performing tasks, going through the motions, but my mind had disconnected.

Scott and I visited our doctor that day to strategize how to get tested without alerting our insurance. In 1990, a positive HIV test could elicit an insurance cancellation with no alternative replacements. He arranged a private test we could pay for in cash to be performed the next day. At the time, there was no definitive HIV test you could take and get the results back within hours. He explained it would take one or two days to receive the results.

Often, in extremely stressful situations in my life, there's some weird sideshow happening that makes me laugh. Well, the day I got my HIV test it was our nurse who provided that moment of comic relief. She started by getting out her notebook from a class she had taken about HIV testing and counseling. Opening it up she read the protocol, word for word. She appeared visibly nervous, continuing through the lengthy notebook in the most awkward way imaginable. Clearly, I was the first person she had ever tested.

I felt bad for her. She was literally shaking. In my heart I rooted for her, trying to make our answers as specific as possible and constantly giving her a reassuring look that she was doing great. Scott and I laughed about the whole scene on the way home. Of course, my insides were numb, heavily in denial ... the thing your body does when you hear bad news and start to think that maybe, just maybe, God will be extra nice to you and somehow, you'll wake up from this dream and go back to life as you knew it.

The next morning the nurse called to confirm. My test

was positive. She said that I should return to the clinic for a more specific test, the Western Blot, to make sure the screening test was not a false positive. She explained that we needed to bring every member of our family in for HIV testing.

Again, my stomach sank to the floor.

Teresa was born before my blood transfusion, but because I had breastfed her, she had a small chance of being infected. Our other two kids, Laura and Ryan, were born to an HIV-positive mother and each had about a 25 percent chance of having contracted the disease from me. Lastly, there was Scott. I'd been pregnant two of the years of my infection, and then Scott had a vasectomy. We hadn't protected ourselves the prior six years from what we didn't know was there. We never once used a condom. Statistically, we were told, Scott had a high chance of being HIV-positive.

Piling into our old Volkswagen Vanagon, we set out to the doctor's office to get our blood drawn. It was Thursday, August 16th. On that drive, looking in the backseat at our kids, my emotions started to kick in. There they were ... my babies ... the three people in the world I would give my life for, my two-year-old, four-year-old, and six-year-old on their way to get tested for a disease that would not only most likely kill them but also that had so much stigma, so much discrimination and baggage connected to it, that I knew it would shatter their innocence. Fighting tears, I looked out the side window, trying my best to keep them from thinking anything was wrong.

I started performing mental gymnastics to remember which one of my kids had been sick the most, which one of them had been the smallest, which one of them had had the most sinus infections, and which one had displayed any kind of sickly look. I kept coming back to Laura. Laura had struggled to gain weight all her four years. She threw up almost everything she ate until she was nine months old, which was attributed to food allergies. Even then, she was only in the fifth percentile in weight. In my mind I just reconciled that Laura was probably infected, and Scott. And, of course, me.

Because we received the results of my first test in one day, I expected the same for my family. Instead, the nurse told us that the lab was closed on Fridays so they would call us on Monday. In *four* days.

We headed home to our almost-empty house with the moving truck sitting out front. Opening the garage, I confronted a mountain of baby goods spilling across the floor. I had thrown it haphazardly into a heap to pass on to the couple who had bought our house. They were expecting their first child. There it all was, lying there, staring at me. Six years of baby paraphernalia taking up almost half of the floor. If these parents knew that we had gone for HIV tests, would they just burn this stuff?

We decided we were going to tell almost nobody about any of this HIV drama. There were so few people we could trust at that point. This was the era of Ryan White, who had died in April of 1990. Only a teenager, he had been in the national headlines for several years, not being allowed to go to school for fear he would spread AIDS.

Also in the news was the Ray family, in Florida. They had three young boys who all had been infected with HIV through blood products for hemophilia. A week after a judge had ordered their school district to allow the boys to attend public school, their house was burned to the ground, and they had to move. These were the stories we followed in the media; there was hardly an article or story about AIDS that wasn't cloaked in fear.

That weekend, waiting for the results, we barely slept. I lost several pounds. Nothing looked appetizing, and nothing tasted right.

I kept thinking, "When I die and Scott dies, who is going to raise our kids?" We had good friends and awesome family members, but I couldn't think of one of them, not one, whom I wanted to raise my kids. I couldn't talk because when I did, I usually ended up crying and I didn't want to let on to the kids that something was seriously wrong. My brain was numb; my heart was broken. Life as we knew it was over. Our world was a mess, that much I knew. I was just waiting until Monday to see how big of a mess it was going to be.

Monday morning finally came. It was supposed to be Scott's first day of work in a new town, three hundred miles away. He called in sick. I'm not sure what he said to get out of work that day, but I am sure it wasn't, "Sorry I can't make it in. We're just sitting here waiting for our HIV tests to come back to see if we have AIDS."

The phone rang. I picked up the receiver and could barely believe the nurse's words: "Everyone in your family is fine, no HIV." I had braced myself for the worst possible news; every muscle in my body was tense and prepared. Tears ran down my face and my body breathed a huge sigh of relief.

But then she added the clincher, "Unfortunately, your second test result came back positive. You are definitely HIV-positive."

Since getting those test results, I've met so many people who are HIV-positive who say that getting their diagnosis was the worst day of their life. But that Monday, I also found out my family, my whole entire family, for some inexplicable reason, was spared this disease. That was such good news it made my own HIV diagnosis not feel so bad in the moment.

I'd survived the worst week of my life, and all I could

think was, "I'll figure this out. I can handle this."

We got in our moving van that afternoon and drove across the state to our new home, three hundred miles away.

IN SICKNESS
AND IN HEALTH

And what's romance?
Usually, a nice little tale where you have everything
as you like it, where the rain never wets your jacket
and gnats never bite your nose.

D.H. Lawrence

grew up going to the Lutheran church. In my younger years, my whole family went to Sunday services and my parents sang in the choir, but sometime around junior high, when my siblings were heading off to college, my parents stopped attending. They often dropped me off by myself for Sunday School and youth groups. I kind of liked church, but I felt like a stranded orphan without my family there.

In high school, church became a place I drove myself on Sunday mornings to relieve my "party guilt" from the night before. As I began college, I started to reflect on faith and God in deeper ways. In the second half of my freshman year, I joined a Bible study, and one of my friends asked me if I wanted to work at a Christian camp during spring break, located in British Columbia, Canada. The camp was owned by a Christian youth outreach organization that mobilized volunteers to mentor high school and middle school students.

Since I didn't have any extra money for a fun trip to

Mexico or Hawaii, where many of my sorority sisters were going for spring break, I said yes to working at the camp, got on the boat in Vancouver, B.C., and headed north.

Even though spring break was in late March, it was thirty-five degrees and raining outside, and I hadn't brought any clothes that were appropriate for freezing cold, almost snowing, temperatures; nonetheless, that week at camp changed the direction of my life.

I never could relate to the evangelical idea of giving my life to God, or letting God into my life, or even becoming a Christian. In fact, everything in me rebelled against any cookie-cutter process as it applied to God. I just felt that I always had God in my life. From the minute I heard, as a young child, about the concept of God, a God who loved me and would take care of me, I just believed that there was such a being. So at camp, at the end of that week, when they asked people to stand up if they wanted to give their life to God, I stayed seated. I figured God already had my life and that he, or she, was already in it.

What changed my life that week was the reality of a Christian community. I liked church but it always seemed like I was at someone else's family reunion. At camp, I began to feel like I belonged.

It changed my life in another way, too. Through my involvement with this outreach organization and its community of college students, I met a young man named Scott. He attended Western Washington University, in Bellingham, while I studied at the University of Washington, ninety miles south in Seattle. I dated a friend of his for a while, whereas he had the same girlfriend the whole four years he was in college. Our connection was our mutual involvement in Christian youth outreach and the community of college students who became our shared friends.

During my senior year in college, Scott and I occasionally ran into each other at camps and events but rarely had a conversation that progressed beyond a greeting. We once double-dated when we were dating other people, but really, there was little interaction outside of our shared youth-leadership interests.

We had no idea that fate would have other plans for us.

A few years after meeting Scott, I'd become a high school science teacher, and my boss, the principal of the school, encouraged me to go back to college and brush up on my physics. The only university offering the courses I needed in the summer of 1981 was Western Washington University, so I ended up temporarily moving to Bellingham. A few days after classes started, I ran into Scott one night at a mutual friend's house, and, lo and behold, we discovered that both of us had moved on from previous relationships and were now single.

In mid-July, Scott showed up at my apartment for our first official date. He'd put a twin mattress in the back of his yellow Chevy Luv pickup, picked up some Kentucky Fried Chicken and a couple of beers, and we set out to watch the sunset on Bellingham Bay. That night my chatty mood got the best of me; I ended up oversharing every detail of my life, good and bad.

When he dropped me off, I thought to myself, "Well, shit, way to divulge every last piece of dirt in your life, you idiot. There's not much he doesn't know. So, I guess he'll either never call me again or he'll ask me to marry him."

Three months later we were engaged, and a year later we were married on Memorial Day weekend in 1982. It was a whirlwind romance.

I quit my teaching job and moved from Seattle to Bellingham the summer we got married. Scott had joined the paid staff of the organization he'd been volunteering for. He was responsible for mentoring and training leaders who volunteered in schools north of Bellingham near the Canadian border. I helped him with this work and had a job at a dentist's office during those early years together. The second year Scott and I were married, we found out we were expecting. In fact, I'm pretty sure I got pregnant on our first anniversary!

At the time, we had done a deep dive into the evangelical church. Now, the thing about evangelicals is they often think that God is speaking to them directly and take the Biblical idea of prophets and prophecy into real time. During my first pregnancy, there were two times when some such person attempted to predict my future or prophesied about my life.

The first was at a Christian retreat put on for women. Twenty-five women sat in a circle, and a lauded guest speaker, known for her wisdom and long, enthusiastic prayers, traveled around the room, placing her hands on each woman's head, and giving them what she said was a "word" or message from God.

Watching her, mesmerized, I sat anxiously waiting my turn, listening to her proclamations for other women. What brilliant piece of direct-from-God wisdom would she have for me? I was hoping for some sort of life-defining divine message. Would these words feel so special they'd send me off on a new life path? Encourage me to greatness? When the inspired speaker finally laid her hands on my head, barely pausing, she whispered, "Get some rest."

That was it. My divine word of encouragement from God. "Get some freaking rest!" I still get a chuckle when I think about it. Either she looked at my pregnant stomach and thought to herself, "Obvious prophecy. Can't go wrong here."

Or ... God is very practical.

The second time something like this happened was that

same fall. Scott had breakfast with a man from our church whom he had just met. While they ate, his new acquaintance explained that God had shown him in a dream that we were destined to have a baby boy. God had told him we were to name him Matthew.

Scott came home and promptly told me, "Well, 1 know what we're NEVER going to name one of our children!"

In March 1984, 1 gave birth to a baby girl, and we named her Teresa after one of the saints, Mother Teresa. Looking back on that now, it's like, "Hey, little baby, we're going to name you after one of the world's most selfless people. Grow up, sell all your possessions, become a nun, and spend your life taking care of people on the streets, dying in India. No pressure!"

My AIDS story started on the day that Teresa was born. 1 spent the night before doing what 1 always did on Monday night: going to the outreach group meeting at Meridian High School as a youth leader. We settled in at home around eleven o'clock, and 1 went to sleep only to wake up in the middle of the night with a distinct feeling that my water had broken. Scott jumped out of bed in our tiny room and flipped on the light expecting to see wet sheets. Instead, when our eyes adjusted to the light, what we saw was a huge pool of blood. This was not what they told me to expect in Lamaze class.

Turning to Scott, 1 noticed his face seemed a bit drained, a little white from the surprise. 1 fetched my bag, already packed for the hospital, and we set out knowing it would never again be just the two of us. As we pulled up to the emergency room, the nurse on duty immediately brought a wheelchair ... to Scott.

1 looked over, pointed to my stomach, and said, "Hello ... I'm the one who's pregnant here."

Scott did look a little ghostly, and the nurse replied to

him, "Well, you'd better sit down and put your head between your legs. Try to get some blood back into that brain of yours."

We went into the delivery area, and I was hooked up to monitors to assess the progress of the delivery. After a few hours, the doctor decided that very little headway had been made and to speed things up, I'd be given an IV of the drug Pitocin. After that, I was in labor for twelve hours with no big complications. We never did get a good answer as to why there had been so much blood when my water broke.

Teresa entered the world at 2:59 that afternoon. I remember exactly what time she was born because the nurse who'd been assisting was ending her shift at 3:00, and she kept saying, "I've put way too much effort into this; we need to get that baby out so I can see if it's a boy or girl!"

I'm not a medical doctor, but my understanding is that the drug, Pitocin, was given to me to help my uterus contract, which speeds up the delivery. Unfortunately, after the delivery, the effects of Pitocin stopped, and my body started hemorrhaging blood. For hours after Teresa was born, nurses massaged my stomach, trying different medications to get my uterus to contract so the hemorrhaging would stop.

So many giant blood clots came out of my body that they gave me a sleeping pill so that I wouldn't get stressed out watching it happen. Scott, on the other hand, the same person who had practically fainted after he saw the initial blood on our bed, was a trooper. He spent hours in my hospital room that night, helping the nurses with this hemorrhage; it was happening fast and there was a ton of blood.

The next day when they raised the head of my hospital bed, I started to lose consciousness and pass out. My doctor informed me that my hematocrit or red blood cell count was very low from the hemorrhage. To get my strength back, I would need a blood transfusion.

That afternoon, on March 14, three units of blood were transfused into my arm to replace the blood I'd lost.

By then I knew about AIDS. I paid attention to the headlines, mostly because HIV was being portrayed as a gay disease, and I have a beloved brother who is gay. I didn't know anything specific about AIDS in 1984 other than that many of the people who were infected with HIV died. I don't remember the disease ever being referred to as HIV at that time; it was always AIDS.

I never, in any way, imagined that AIDS was something that would happen to me. When I got my blood transfusion, it didn't once cross my mind that the blood I received could be infected with HIV. I am, however, surprised that not one medical professional mentioned a risk when I received that blood. It was widely known at that time, in the medical community, that HIV was in the blood supply and that it could be passed through transfusions.

After three days in the hospital hooked up to IVs, I went home with our new baby. I soon went back to work at the dental office. Life was good. Scott continued his career as a director of youth ministries. We had two more kids, and in 1986 we moved to Puyallup, Washington, for a different job with the same organization.

That was it. At least, that's what I thought.

UNEXPLAINABLE SYMPTOMS

I already want to take a nap tomorrow.

Anonymous

A year before I got "the phone call," I started to realize that something was very wrong with me. After having three kids, I quit teaching because the amount of money required for three young kids to be in daycare exceeded what I made as a teacher. Nonetheless, Scott and I needed extra income, so I looked for an evening job when Scott could be at home with the kids. I ended up working as a waitress, Monday through Thursday, at a nice Italian restaurant in South Seattle. I'd waitressed in college, and I really did enjoy any job where you could walk out the door at the end of the night with a hundred dollars in your pocket from tips.

That fall, I began to feel unusually sick. I went to several doctors, and I would tell them that I was having some recurring symptoms: I was easily exhausted, I often felt weak, I kept getting swollen glands, and I was occasionally sweating at night. Every time I went in for answers there would be a battery of tests. When I'd return for those results, the same story would replay, over and over.

Each doctor, each time, would look at me and say, "All of the tests that we ran are normal. You're in good health!"

Even though these ailments were classic symptoms of HIV infection, and even though on every medical history form at all of those doctors' offices I had checked the box saying that I had a blood transfusion in 1984—a clear risk for HIV infection—no one, not one health professional, thought to run an HIV test. Later, I asked a few of those clinicians, "Why?"

Each one said the same thing, "You just didn't look like someone who would have AIDS."

If you didn't live through the 1980s, you might ask yourself, "What does someone with AIDS look like or what were they supposed to look like?" In 1989, almost everyone who had AIDS was a gay man or an injection drug user. The connection of HIV with the blood supply was getting stronger as physicians became more aware that much of the hemophiliac population had been infected through blood products they received to clot blood.

A white, heterosexual, young mom was not what they were looking for, even when her history and symptoms matched this infection.

The only person who ever suggested that maybe I was infected with HIV was my mom. One day, that same year, while I was at her house telling her about all of my symptoms, she said, "Well, you know, you did have that blood transfusion. Has anyone ever tested you for AIDS?"

My response to her was quick and brief: "Mom, I don't have AIDS."

And then, "Please don't go telling the relatives that I do."

My mom had a tendency that if she thought of something long enough, she would actually convince herself that it was happening and that it was true. I shut that down as fast as possible. The truth was, I really didn't want to consider being infected with HIV, so I just waved it off as quickly as I could and forgot about it.

At the time she mentioned this, I was very aware of how HIV was spread. I knew that some people had been infected with HIV through the blood supply. But still, most of the people that I saw or read about who were dying of AIDS were gay men. So, like my doctors, I didn't think that it was something that would happen to me. I worried about my brother but was in no way worrying about myself in this context. When Mom mentioned HIV as something I should consider, it was so unthinkable to me that I decided, consciously, to just not think about it.

I'd been feeling so crummy that I quit my waitressing job, even though I loved it. Suffering from a terrible cold and a sinus infection, I'd felt so rundown that I told my boss, "I don't think I can do this; I'm exhausted."

The restaurant owner, the sweetest guy, supportively urged, "Please, please don't quit. Why don't you just take a week off and rest?"

So, Scott and I planned a getaway to a friend's cabin on the water.

As soon as we arrived at this cozy little retreat, I fell asleep. And by "fell asleep," I mean I slept for three days. A couple of times during that weekend, Scott got so worried that he came into the bedroom or over to the sofa and checked on me to make sure I was still breathing. I simply could not wake up. I can only think that my immune system was so shot that sleeping and breathing were all it had the energy to do.

In January 1990, we kicked off the year by going to a Christian staff conference in San Diego. While enjoying the sun in Southern California, our Regional Director began talking to us about a great opportunity for Scott to direct their work and programs in Spokane. This possibility interested both of us because we'd been raised in Central Washington and missed the weather on that side of the

Cascade mountains. To say it more simply, we were sick of the Seattle-area rain.

We traveled to Spokane in May, and Scott interviewed for the position and was offered the job. This was the reason we were moving when we got the call.

The call that changed everything about what would happen when we moved to Spokane.

CHRIS

I smile because you're my brother.
I laugh because there's nothing you can do
about it.

Unknown Author

My original family, the one I was born into, consisted of two parents and four kids. I was the caboose, the baby—four years younger than my three siblings, who are all a year apart. I was the surprise, born after my parents were "done" having children. My dad used to sum it up by saying that "I was the best mistake he ever made."

My relationships with my brothers and sister varied. Being younger, I didn't have many points of connection with the older two. I was in grade school while they were living out their high school years. But my brother Chris, the third-born, actually seemed to enjoy being with me. As far back as I can remember, Chris was a constant and loving presence in my life. Even though he was a boy and older, he put up with me and often gave the impression that he even liked his little sister. I felt accepted by him. We told each other almost everything. He even filled me in on where babies come from. When we got into trouble together, he usually took the blame.

I have so many happy memories with Chris. A set of wooden dollhouse furniture he gave me that he whittled himself. Sitting under a dock together overseas, eating sticky buns and watching the fish swim by. The white sweater he bought me at the airport, a surprise just because I'd liked it. My big brother. I had taken his throne as the baby of the family, and he had allowed it and loved me anyway. We did things most kids just dream about doing but are wise enough to leave in their imaginations.

One of our favorite and most laughed-about stunts was when we lived in the Marshall Islands where my dad was superintendent of schools for a few years. The island was tiny, and there wasn't much in the way of entertainment for kids, so we came up with some very creative ways to pass an afternoon. The small phone book on the island listed residents' phone numbers and where they worked. One woman, Betty Ross, had a strong Southern accent that sixth-grade Chris could mimic perfectly. So one day, Chris called every wife from the company Betty's husband worked for and invited them to a tea party at her house. Women were asking, "What should I bring?" and he didn't miss a beat, offering suggestions. Unfortunately, the party was planned for a time when we were in school, so we never saw if it came to fruition. It was one time, a rare occasion in our childhood, that we didn't get caught. Although we did confess to our parents some twenty years later.

Chris was a kid with a huge heart, an active imagination, and somehow, always a steady stream of cash coming his way. In so many ways we have always been opposites. When we were young, I was skinny and he was stocky. In junior high, I was the straight-A cheerleader, and he was the kid who could not be done with high school fast enough, accumulating enough credits to graduate several months early. In college, I was the sorority blonde while he was becoming the first male phone operator in Seattle. We lived in two totally different worlds but always with a bond that defied our differences.

When the nurse called and confirmed I had HIV, my first inclination wasn't to call Chris. Instead, I called my sister, Claudia. As an adult, I'm close to my only sister and she has worked in healthcare her whole life, so I thought she could help me navigate this new world of AIDS with her medical connections. But when I gave her the details, her only response was, "Have you told Chris?" And then again, "You need to call and tell Chris."

My brother Chris is a gay man, and by 1990 he'd lost several of his friends to AIDS. Many of his friends were either sick or dying so I had asked him a few times, "Are you HIV-positive?"

His answer was always, "Don't worry about me, I'm just fine."

I knew his response wasn't exactly, "No, I don't have AIDS," so part of me always assumed that maybe, or probably, he was HIV-positive.

So that day, I told Chris, "You know, I had that blood transfusion after Teresa was born, and as it turns out I was infected with HIV."

Quietly and slowly, he responded, "Well, to tell you the truth, I'm in the same boat."

Chris explained that he'd been diagnosed four years earlier and was doing pretty well since starting the only AIDS drug available, AZT.

"So," I asked, "what did Mom and Dad say?"

"I haven't told them." He paused. "I'm not going to tell them."

At that point, the only person in our family he had told about his diagnosis was my sister. I began to wrap my head around all of the reasons why Chris would not want to tell my parents. At the same time, I was trying to reconcile that with all of the reasons I needed and wanted to tell them. I couldn't imagine dealing with a potentially fatal disease and not having my parents there to support not only me, but my family. Was I being insensitive? This was no longer just about me, and I certainly didn't want a bunch of attention and focus from my parents while none was going toward Chris.

I took a step back in my mind and thought, "We can talk about this later."

All I said back to him was, "I might need to tell them, but I'm certainly not going to tell them about me without telling them about you."

My brother single-handedly took over my care at that point. Scott had gone on to Spokane to start his new job. The kids were with his parents, whom we had hastily told what was going on out of necessity. I had no idea what to do next. I wasn't sure whom I wanted to tell this to, what doctor I wanted to go to, how to figure out the extent of damage to my immune system, and where, exactly, to find care and information. I stayed in Seattle with Chris, not knowing if Spokane would have the same resources I knew my brother had access to.

Chris accompanied me to the Northwest AIDS Foundation, an agency of social service providers solely dedicated to acting as liaisons between people living with HIV and available care services, or, to put it simply, people helping infected individuals navigate the world of AIDS. I met with a case manager, a lovely, calm, and reassuring woman who handed me a pile of pamphlets and enough information to spin my head. She said that I needed to get my T-cell count, which would tell me a lot about the state of my immune system. I didn't even know what a T cell was at that point, but I did remember that the nurse who gave me the initial HIV test had also drawn blood and said I could call her for my baseline counts. I assumed that included the ever-so-important T cells.

I hung out with my brother for a couple of days, and because he was talking calmly about HIV and AIDS, and because he had so much experience and knew friends who were infected, many living fairly normal lives, I began to feel reassured, like maybe this wouldn't be so bad.

One of the things I thought about every day was the fear of infecting Scott. Not only would I kill the love of my life, but also the man I was hoping would stay alive and raise our kids. Chris calmed some of those fears. I learned that it is actually harder for a woman to infect a man with HIV than it is for a man to infect a woman. It makes sense when you think that all the sexual parts of a woman are internal, and the virus tends to be inside a woman longer. But, of course, this was not a one-night stand—it was six years of intimacy.

Chris and I were wandering through downtown Seattle, walking around a shopping area, admiring a small Chihuly glass exhibit. I decided to call the nurse to get my T-cell count. Next to a Bank of America by the entrance to the shops stood a row of pay phones. I picked up the receiver on one and dialed her number. She let me know that I had 425 T cells.

That's where I started ... my baseline of sorts. When I told this to Chris, he said, "That's good ... that's really, really good."

Chris explained that with a count over two hundred, I was just considered HIV-positive. To get an official AIDS diagnosis, you either had to have a CD4 (T-cell) count of less than two hundred, or an infection that was an opportunistic infection on the list of AIDS-defining conditions put out by the CDC. They were always updating that list and, at that time, didn't have symptoms specific to women.

I was so thankful to have one person whom I could

walk with through this nightmare. Someone who was experiencing the same things physically but who had so much more information. Someone I could trust completely. Chris understood the degree of "tired" I was feeling and the confusion and fear in looking toward the future. He added in a joke now and then about this stupid disease, which made me laugh and reminded me I could, indeed, still laugh.

It saddened me that my brother had to deal with this horrible disease, AIDS, but part of me also felt extremely comforted by the assurance that I was not alone.

I guess misery really does love company.

DR. C

Everyone wants to go to heaven,
but nobody wants to die.

Unknown Author

My sister, Claudia, set me up with a doctor in Spokane who was a pulmonologist. She had known him from a hospital in Seattle where she worked in the pulmonary function lab. What I really needed was an infectious disease physician, but I liked the idea of going to someone who one of us knew. Claudia made the appointment with his office in the first week I'd be in Spokane.

I was nervously looking forward to this appointment. Chris told me that there was only one HIV drug available, AZT, and encouraged me to start taking it as soon as possible. I made my way to the 5th and Browne medical building in Spokane and checked in with the receptionist at Dr. C's office.

In the years to follow, Dr. C and I became friends. One year, his family went to British Columbia with us on vacation. But on the day I met him, the day of my first-ever "I have HIV" doctor appointment, Dr. C presented himself as a serious, almost clinical to a fault, non-emotional young clinician. There was little in the way of a sympathetic bedside manner except a brief mention, while he was reading my chart, that "Wow! You could be MY wife."

I will forever remember the first two questions Dr. C asked me: Do you have a living will? Are your things in order?

My brain digested and pondered, "What thirty-two-year-old has a living will? Obviously, one who is going to die soon."

Shaken and a bit out of body, I could hear myself ask, "How long do you think I have to live?"

"Well"—he looked awkwardly toward the ceiling—"maybe three to five years? But, the last two years you'll be very sick, so do anything you want to do as soon as possible."

I left the parking lot at the 5th and Browne in a daze. I began to contemplate what to do with the "three to five." My eyes filled with tears ... and then the parking attendant said, "That'll be a quarter."

I looked at him for clarification. "You mean twenty-five cents?"

"Yes."

For a minute I was distracted completely, being so used to the expensive parking in Seattle and wondering to myself, "How in the world does this guy get a paycheck?"

Then I cried hysterically the rest of the way to our apartment.

SHAG RUG

*It is during our darkest moments
that we must focus to see the light.*

Aristotle

Spokane, Washington: second largest city in the state, childhood home of Bing Crosby, the inventors of Father's Day, and, as of Labor Day, 1990, home of the Lewis Family.

Labor Day on the South Hill is festive with a large Spokane Symphony concert in Manito Park every year. We drove into town around dinnertime with absolutely no knowledge of the concert, picked up fast food at Zip's Drive-In, and proceeded to find a spot to eat. The streets overflowed with parked cars for the concert, so we ended up in a grade school parking lot and our kids rotated between eating their hamburgers and playing on the playground.

About a month before our arrival, we'd bought a house on the South Hill, a house nicer than any we had ever owned, situated around the corner from a brand-new grade school due to open that fall. Unfortunately, the house would not be vacated by the current owners until Halloween, which forced us into a variety of temporary housing situations for a couple of months. That first night, the night before Teresa's first day of first grade, we stayed at a downtown hotel, Cavanaugh's. The next morning, I realized I needed to make her lunch for school, and although we had bought some food the night before, well, I'll just say, it is hard to make a peanut butter sandwich with no utensils—but it can be done!

We moved from the hotel to an apartment that would be our "home" until we'd be able to settle into our new house at the end of October.

Before I describe our temporary living space, the apartment, let me just preface by adding that in the '90s, it was very hard to find any kind of affordable housing that would rent to you on a month-to-month contract. This was long before the days of Airbnb, and we were lucky to find any kind of two-bedroom situation for only two months. Having said that, let me do my best to describe this apartment we moved into.

I don't remember exactly how we got the apartment, and I don't remember how our furniture got into this apartment. In fact, there are a lot of things about those weeks that I just don't remember. But I do remember the darkness of the ground floor, the early 1970s mid-century look, and not in a throwback kind of way but in a "was never redecorated in the last thirty years" kind of way. Olive green seemed to be the predominant color, complete with the ever-so-awesome shag carpet popular in my childhood.

The two-bedroom apartment put the girls in one room and left Ryan sleeping on the floor of our bedroom. The one saving grace, the one truly awesome thing about this depressingly dark and musty basement apartment, was that it came with an indoor swimming pool. I don't think the kids cared about anything once they saw that they had a place with a pool! I rarely ever swam in the two months we lived there, but almost every day, when Scott got home from work, he took the kids swimming so I could rest.

That apartment is where I first started taking AZT. I was

to take five pills a day, exactly four hours apart. Chris told me that when he first started taking AZT, he had to take six pills, but the doctors soon decided to forgo the middle-of-the-night pill, to not interrupt sleep. I was provided a pill container with a timer set to beep every four hours. It was critical not to miss a pill because my body could build up resistance to the medication, causing it to stop working effectively.

Every time that timer went off, I was reminded: I would be taking pills for the rest of my life.

And that life would be over in three to five years.

RYAN AND THE MILK

*The most important thing in illness
is never lose heart.*

Nikolai Lenin

ZT hit me like a bulldozer. It knocked me out. I came around, conscious, every few hours to totally barf up everything I'd eaten. Exhausted, and shaking all the time, I fought off chills and headaches, all while trying to absorb my short life expectancy.

My mind sort of tabled the long-term thinking to simply survive each hour. I was the sickest I'd ever been in my life. At the same time, I still had to take care of three small kids. Scott was constantly working, trying to be stellar in his brand-new job. The last thing we needed was for him to have a problem, like AIDS discrimination, and lose our health insurance and income. I was certainly in no condition to go to work.

We tried to be as confidential as possible, retreating into the closet of silence and secrecy regarding my health. Besides Chris and Claudia, only a few close family members knew about the diagnosis, along with a couple of Scott's colleagues since our health insurance was being run through their main office in Colorado Springs. All of those people lived at least three hundred miles away, so my world shrank dramatically.

Upon arrival to our new city, I knew one person in Spokane: Kristine. She'd been my sorority sister in college, never a best friend, more like a very close acquaintance. In our younger years we never hung out with the same people, probably because she was in the next class and really, Kristine often felt like she was several years older than me. But at that moment, there were two things I knew for sure. One was that Kristine took care of everyone and everything in our college days—she was an excellent caregiver— and the second thing I was certain of was that I desperately needed care.

So, I called Kristine, explaining our situation. I didn't have the luxury of extra time to catch up naturally and lean into this private conversation. I just rang her up after several years of absence and regurgitated the whole HIV saga on our first chat. She, being the boss caregiver I remembered from college, never wavered or flinched, never seemed worried for herself or phased by the stigma or fear of AIDS. She just sprang into action.

First, she enrolled Laura in a prestigious preschool. The class roster had been completely full for months, but Kristine worked her magic and somehow got Laura in. During those first couple of months in Spokane, she brought us food, she listened to me, she gave me hugs at a time when it seemed only Princess Diana was willing to hug someone with AIDS, and she prayed for me every day. She was my one friend.

When classes started in September, on most days, Scott would take Teresa to the grade school, and Kristine would show up at our apartment a little later to pick up Laura for preschool because her son was in the same class. After everyone departed, almost always it was only Ryan and me hanging out together. On these days I laid low, doing as little as possible, basically being a semi-functioning parent while hoping to make it to the bathroom if I was sick.

Lying on the couch one morning after the girls left for school, I was very sick. I looked across the room at my two-

and-a-half-year-old who had gotten his own bowl out of the cupboard, climbed up on the counter, retrieved a box of Life cereal, and then proceeded to open the refrigerator, and drag out the milk. I'm not talking about a small carton of milk; being a family of five, milk only showed up by the gallon. There he was, my tiny little guy, balancing a gallon of milk on his stomach as he carried it across the room, and dumped it into his cereal bowl, like a mini tsunami, spilling everything everywhere. He then commenced eating his breakfast.

During this whole scene I, his mom and caregiver, lay on the couch observing, as though paralyzed. I couldn't move. Frozen on the sofa, my body so nauseated and exhausted that I couldn't respond other than to watch.

At that moment, I felt a deep sense of failure. I felt defeated. I could see my own death playing out before me along with the realization that all of this would take a great toll on my kids.

As I kept taking AZT, my body fought against the drug with everything it had. One evening Chris called. I'd been vomiting right before so I was literally outside the bathroom door lying on the shag carpet in the hall. Phone in hand, eyes shut, trying to get through the conversation without having to return to the toilet, I told him, "I just don't think I can do this. I don't think I can tolerate this medicine."

I'll never forget what he said to me that night. I'm even willing to say that he might've saved my life.

"You have to take the medicine. You can't stop taking the medicine," he pleaded. "People who stop taking the medicine die."

Chris then continued to explain to me that, usually, if you keep taking the pills, eventually your body gets used to them and you tolerate the side effects more and more. But, he added, "This could take a couple of months."

That's exactly what ended up happening.

I'll forever think of those two months, living in the olive-green basement apartment, as some of the darkest days of my life. I'm somewhat grateful for that apartment, because, by the time we moved into our South Hill house on Halloween, the side effects from AZT had lessened.

When we closed the door to that basement, I left behind the initial despair and the worst of the AZT side effects, along with the shag carpet and the all-too-familiar bathroom floor.

DR. WINTERS

*Real knowledge is to know the extent
of one's ignorance.*

Confucius

990 was the third year in Washington State that public schools were required to have AIDS education, starting in the fifth grade. During the first month of classes, a flier went out saying that there would be a parent night to discuss the AIDS curriculum. This obviously interested me even though Teresa was just a first grader.

Trying to appear as put-together as I could, despite my exhaustion, I joined all the other parents, looking like giants awkwardly perched on child-sized chairs in the school's auditorium. An administrator from the school district and a nurse presented the required lessons for each grade level, not only for grade school but also what would be required and taught in middle school and high school. This came to be known as the KNOW curriculum. I was very interested, not only because this AIDS thing had become my life and, at this point, I was still learning about HIV myself, but also because I was a trained high school science/health educator; I was curious about what they were teaching.

After the presentation, the nurse asked if there were any questions or concerns. It was then that one of the parents raised his hand, stood up, and confidently began talking.

"Hello, l am Dr. Winters, a medical doctor. I've been following the AIDS epidemic very closely. l have seen the conclusions from the CDC and the National Institutes of Health, and l just want to say that l don't trust these findings."

l felt myself shrinking into my small plastic chair.

He continued, "l think it's really too soon in this disease to know all of the ways that the virus is contracted. l think we should be very cautious and not underestimate that there could be several other ways that this infection is spread."

At that point, l stopped listening and just watched the wave of concern pass over the sea of parents. What had started as a matter-of-fact explanation of the new curriculum, just as mundane as if we'd been discussing spelling or multiplication, became something more, something to fear, all from one man's thoughts. He was, after all, a doctor.

Well, thank you, fucking Dr. Winters. You just, single-handedly, solidified strongly in my mind that there was no way l was telling any of these people that l had HIV.

l went home that night sinking deeper and deeper into depression and isolation.

l cried myself to sleep one more time.

PARENTS

When sorrows like sea billows roll.

Horatio Gates Spafford

We'd stopped in Yakima on the way to Spokane while moving in August and shared my diagnosis with Scott's parents, Mel and Eleanor. They, of course, were blown away. Both of them had very little knowledge of AIDS, so, to the best of my ability, I explained to them what I knew about the disease and also told them I was going to the doctor soon and would have a lot more information after that.

Scott's parents stepped up to help us in many ways, but Mel and Eleanor were not my parents. As much as they loved me, and I knew they did, I wasn't their daughter.

I knew telling them about my illness was a walk in the park compared to what it was going to be like to tell my own parents.

Dick and Coyet, my mom and dad, grew up in the Depression, fell in love in college, and got married young. They created a family in the early 1950s, three kids in three years, Curt, Claudia, and Chris. Then, four years later, after they were all finished having kids, along came Julie. And yes, I always wondered why I didn't get a "C" name like the rest of the crew.

My dad was a high school teacher, a high school principal, and, eventually, a superintendent of schools. He loved kids, and because of that, he was an easygoing and fun parent to have around. My friends loved my dad; he was a sensitive, caring, and affectionate parent.

Mom, on the other hand, grew up in a family with an alcoholic father. She contracted polio as a young girl and had to go to North Carolina to recover while living with her grandparents. Her sister was one year older than her and very popular in school. The way my mom explains it, she was often the caregiver for her younger sister and brother because her mother got cancer and ended up dying before I was born. She always painted her childhood in a somewhat dismal way.

My mom showed her love for the four of us kids by doing things for us. She worked hard at her various jobs, she was a very good cook, with dinner waiting for us every night promptly at six o'clock, she sewed a lot of our clothes, she planted gardens, and she drove us around to all our activities. Mom definitely believed that men were superior to women. In her view, women were here to serve. She lived this out but also complained about it most of her life. The most difficult thing about Mom, especially when I was young, was that she was not the most affectionate person. Her favor came only when her children performed, when we did something she approved of. There weren't many hugs; there wasn't much praise. She was often difficult to please.

All that is to say, my dad was my "go-to" person when it came to anything relational or emotional. Really, he was my preferred parent when it came to almost anything.

I'd say, in many ways, I experienced a different relationship with my parents than the other kids in our family. Being the youngest, the add-on, the unexpected fourth child, I've often been viewed by my siblings as the "spoiled child." Curt,

Claudia, and Chris, the three "C's," reminded me constantly that I was the recipient of many things and privileges they didn't have or enjoy.

In those years, when it was just Mom, Dad, and me, my parents were more like partners, even friends. My dad and I used to go on a lot of drives, escaping Mom's mood swings. A favorite of ours was to hit up Dairy Queen—he loved the Peanut Buster Parfaits. Dad and I spent a ton of time together, and I always thought that I had a special relationship with him. I'd come to find out, as an adult, that somehow he'd created that sense in every one of his kids. We all thought we were his favorite in some way.

So, as you can imagine, the thought of telling my parents, especially Dad, that two of their kids were living with a fatal illness was the last thing I wanted to do, and yet it was the most important thing I needed in my life as I tried to figure out how to manage AIDS and prepare to possibly die soon.

I desperately needed my dad.

It was February 1991. I'd known that I was HIV-positive for about six months, and I was really having a hard time lying to my parents about how my life was going. I had been begging Chris to tell them.

He finally said, "You can tell them, but I really don't want to be there."

I didn't blame him; I didn't want to be there either.

The moment arrived on Presidents' Day weekend, which was also Scott's birthday. I called Mom and Dad earlier in the week and told them that we were going to make the seven-hour drive from Spokane to Hood Canal to visit them. I also said that we wouldn't be bringing our kids, that we were going to drop them off in Yakima at Scott's parent's house on the way to see them.

My dad asked, "Why?"

All I said back was, "Well, we have something kind of important we want to talk to you about."

What a terrible thing to do to your parents. I would have hated that. Later, Dad would tell me that he and my mom sat for hours brainstorming what it could be that would be so traumatic or private that we would need to leave our kids at Scott's parents before coming to talk to them. He told me that they finally concluded that we were probably coming to tell them we were getting divorced.

It was a long, nerve-racking drive to the Canal. I was rehearsing in my mind exactly how to present this to them. I knew it would be devastating news. When we arrived at their house, the sun was setting, and I wasted no time getting right to the point of the trip. We were all sitting in the living room. Scott and I were on the couch, Dad was in a chair on the other side of the room, and Mom was moving between the kitchen and the living room, eventually coming around and sitting in another chair.

Right off Dad asked, "Well, what do you want to talk to us about?"

I felt the saliva drain from my throat, but I tried to start talking anyway. After about three words, I teared up; there was a lump blocking my vocal cords and no words would come.

At that point, Scott took over. He started to talk to my dad and mom and gave them the sad news that two of their kids had HIV and the prognosis was not great.

When he started to talk about my blood transfusion, Mom said, "I just knew it." That was the last thing she said before she got up and went to the bathroom. She didn't come out for a couple of hours.

Dad, on the other hand, instantly shifted into a very professional, superintendent-of-school kind of demeanor with a guarded and in-control voice. He asked questions about HIV, wondering if there were any hopeful treatments. He wanted to know all about my doctor and various things like that.

And then he said something that I'll never forget. Something that no one else has ever said to me since. Dad looked me in the eye and said, "You're going to beat this."

Then he held me, and we had quite a good cry.

My mom came out of the bathroom in the early evening and commenced making dinner. She never said a word about any of this the rest of the weekend. As I was leaving on Sunday, she said, "I wish you hadn't moved to Spokane." That was it.

In fact, my mom didn't say a word to me about AIDS for two more years; she never really wanted to have a conversation about it. I wondered about that off and on. I don't know—maybe, just like me, she wanted to say something, but the words wouldn't come.

Later, Dad talked to me about how hard it was to carry this AIDS burden, this giant weight that two of his kids were really sick, and yet not be able to tell anyone about it. When they finally did tell their friends, oftentimes, people would ask how I was doing but wouldn't ask about my brother. It felt like they were insinuating that I didn't deserve to have this disease, that I was an innocent victim, but that Chris, a gay man, wasn't worthy of their sympathy.

This broke my dad's heart. It broke mine, too.

THREE TO FIVE

*Faith consists in believing when it is beyond
the power of reason to believe.*

Voltaire

S ince going to the doctor, the one thing I thought about most was, "What do I do with the three to five years I have left to live?"

Little things started happening that highlighted the fact that I wasn't expected to be around after 1995. One conversation with my siblings in September of 1990, about our parents' fortieth wedding anniversary, reminded me, once again, my life was a ticking time bomb.

I remember the four of us sitting together and I asked my brothers and sister, "So, what should we do for Mom and Dad's fortieth?"

This began a long discussion with one of them reminding me that I had just moved to Spokane and was in transition and that everyone had a lot going on. Then my older brother and sister suggested that we just wait and throw them a big party for their fiftieth wedding anniversary.

The "three to five" popped into my mind instantly, and I gave a glance to Chris. He looked at me, doing sort of a side smirk. I didn't need to say anything to him because the truth was, neither of us expected to be alive in the year 2000 for the big fiftieth celebration.

In my mind, I thought, "Well, good luck with that party."

Scott and I decided that we should have a will drawn up before I died. We also needed to have legal guardians for the kids in case, for some reason, we both died. The first people we asked to be legal guardians to our children were very good friends of ours. A few days after we brought it up, they got back to us and said that they'd thought about it, and had decided it would be too much for them to take on three more kids with the two they already had.

I have to admit, I was a little shocked. I guess it never occurred to me that someone would say no. But then, I was also glad that they had thought enough about it to give us an honest answer. Had we been two healthy parents, they probably would have said yes without a second thought, assuming the worst wouldn't happen. We ended up having Scott's dad be not only the executor of our estate, but also the legal guardian of the kids. Scott and I told his dad that he could decide, depending on our kids' ages, where he thought it would be best for the kids to live. I'm not sure if we "passed the buck" on that decision or not, but, at the time, it seemed to make sense.

Every day I'd see healthy moms; I'd jealously ponder how lucky they were that they would see their kids get out of grade school, that they would be able to teach them to drive, that they would be able to go to their high school graduations, send them off to college, help them plan their weddings, and maybe even someday have grandchildren. None of that was in my plans with the "three to five."

The truth was, not only did I anticipate not being at my kids' high school graduations, but I wasn't even expecting to see them get out of grade school. On the three-year plan, I wouldn't even see Ryan start first grade. If I lived only three years, it meant that my children would be motherless at five, seven, and nine years old.

In my everyday life, the "three to five" was what made me tear up at any given time of any given day. I was grieving the life I wouldn't have and the life my children would experience without me.

Waiting to die. It was a terrible way to live.

I found myself in the midst of a dark, numb sadness. The smallest tasks were exhausting. To get through the day, I broke everything down to the tiniest components, focusing only on one responsibility at a time. Things like getting dressed, cleaning my house, going to the grocery store, or cooking a meal felt like mountains to climb. It took deliberate and concentrated effort. Some days I succeeded in looking almost normal. Many days I dressed only to go back to bed. Sometimes I cried all day. Many nights I lay awake sobbing in my pillow. There were long stretches of no feelings at all, nothing but numbness.

And then came the most dreadful thought of all: I began to wonder if this darkness, this sadness, this depression, was permanent. How would I go on in this heaviness? For the first time in my life, I began to understand suicide. I don't remember ever thinking of ending my life, but I do remember thinking that I didn't want to go on forever in this pain.

My sadness stretched on for months, and then one day I woke up and thought, "You know, I don't feel any more dead today than I did five months ago."

I don't know if it was a conscious decision or not, but something just happened, something changed. I began to slip very deeply into denial. I've read about the stages of grief, and I went through many of those phases, but denial was something I leaned on for a number of years. Part of that denial was imagining that I wasn't going to die.

I would talk about my future life like I expected to live a long time; I began to imagine a longer time span. I wrote about this change in my journal in 1992:

> I try to believe and hope that a long, healthy life could be true for me. I often imagine lots of time with my kids. I tell them what a good grandma I'm going to be and how I'm going to spoil their kids. It's fun to watch them imagine me as an old grandma. We always laugh when I say things like that. I've thought about not talking about the future with my kids; I used to feel like it was sort of a lie. Now I've decided that talking about the future is rather helpful and feels hopeful.

Even if all of those things were never going to happen, imagining them was better than nothing at all.

A BOX OF GLOVES

Gratitude is not only the greatest of virtues,
but the parent of all others.

Marcus Tullius Cicero

The Thanksgiving after my diagnosis, my oldest brother, Curt, and his wife came to stay with us in Spokane. We'd never been especially close so just the fact that he was driving five hours to cook us Thanksgiving dinner was a sure indication that I was, indeed, expected to die soon.

I was thrilled to have my brother, who is a professional chef, preparing our Thanksgiving dinner. That holiday, he taught me how to make cranberry sauce from fresh cranberries, something that I've been doing ever since. Curt had brought his giant knife set, a lemon zester, and a few other handy tools that he knew my kitchen would be lacking. It was fun to see him in action. And then something happened that really set me back. He brought out a large box of plastic gloves.

Curt explained that his restaurant was now using plastic gloves at all times to prepare food because of AIDS. He said that not only would they ensure that the food would not get contaminated if someone making it had a blood-borne disease, but also, if the preparer of the food had a compromised immune system, the gloves would protect that person from getting bacteria in their body from raw meat juices or uncooked food that might be unsafe. He'd brought a huge, restaurant-supply-sized box of plastic gloves to leave with me and told me that I could wear them every time I cooked to keep myself healthy and to keep any HIV blood from getting into the food.

There it was. I didn't know what to say. I knew a lot of what he said was probably true, and I'm pretty sure that the health department advised this. But how this felt, for me, was painful. It was a clear reminder that I was not okay, a reminder that I was a threat of some kind, not only to Thanksgiving dinner, but to anyone and everyone. It wasn't my brother's fault at all; he was trying to help, attempting to calm my fears of infecting my family and my fears of getting sicker. He was sincere and loved me. I knew this, and still, all I felt in that moment was damaged and sad on a Thanksgiving Day where it was becoming harder and harder to be thankful.

PRETENDING

The worst crime is faking it.
Kurt Cobain

I was thinking that I really needed to weave into this dialogue some of the good things that were happening to our family in 1990. In reality, the whole "AIDS thing" was a sideshow we were hiding while our lives continued to move forward.

The kids were making friends. Our new neighbors were amazing from day one. When we moved into our house on Halloween, Laura had pneumonia so she couldn't trick-or-treat. One of the moms in the neighborhood, who had a little girl the same age, split up all of her Halloween candy and brought half of it to Laura. I'd just met her that very day. This was a taste of the next few years and the many ways our neighbors would become like extended family.

In those first six months, Scott was thriving at his new job. It was like he was made for Spokane and the youth-ministries work there. Because Scott's job had its own community, interacting daily with a variety of people was one of the perks of the job. Scott was mentoring twenty to thirty youth leaders who were working with kids in about ten schools and Whitworth College; he also led the local adult advisory committee.

In the meantime, I'd become an incredibly gifted liar. Being a person of faith and still subject to a fair amount of guilt in the lying department, I got proficient at the half truth, giving just enough truth in the lie that it almost seemed like there was no lie at all.

It was pretty easy to excuse myself from anything because "I have three little kids who constantly make me tired and busy," or, "The kids need me for some mom time."

If I looked tired, I could say, "I slept terribly," or, "I'm working hard getting the house together," or, "I have a cold with this change of climate," or, "I have new allergies over here on the Eastside," or, "I'm getting these weird headaches—must be all of the new things."

None of these things were completely false, but they weren't the real reason I was not showing up. Hiding my life was exhausting and required a lot of excuses. It was pretty easy to lie, but it made me feel very hollow on the inside and was a major roadblock to any real friendship or intimacy.

Despite my best efforts to cover up my illness, people were noticing that I wasn't attending meetings and events. But nobody, I mean, absolutely not one person was ever thinking, "I bet she has AIDS!"

In the 1990s, the wife of a youth-ministries-area director was viewed kind of like a pastor's wife. I'd say to Scott, "Well, they think they're getting a two for one," and in a way they were. Because, like a pastor's wife, I was expected to participate in the ministry but not receive my own compensation. There was a strong cultural preference in this Christian community, at the time, that a mother's place was in the home, raising her family and helping her husband.

Nobody ever challenged any of our excuses about my involvement until one day an older woman on Scott's Board, Beverly, started asking questions.

She confronted Scott: "You know, in your interview we were so impressed with Julie because of her past work as a leader and a mentor to other women leaders. We also loved how you both worked as a team. I've been surprised that we haven't seen more of her. Is something wrong?"

Beverly was definitely on to something, so Scott and I decided to tell her and her husband the truth. One night we got a babysitter and went to their house to have a chat. We sat in their living room, and Scott proceeded to tell this lovely couple our AIDS story.

What happened next was a new level of "WTF? How do I even respond to this?"

Beverly and her husband were quiet the whole time Scott talked about my diagnosis, sitting together on their floral loveseat across from us, their faces blank, giving away nothing. Then we were all silent for a few minutes after he finished—an awkward silence where I found myself staring at my hands to avoid accidental eye contact, all the while very aware of a ticking clock that seemed to grow louder with each second.

Suddenly, Beverly broke the silence. Very matter-of-factly, as if she'd come up with the solution to it all, she said, "Let's just pretend it's cancer."

I want to make it very clear that I have all the sympathy in the world for anyone who is dealing with cancer or with any disease, especially one that could be fatal. Beverly was probably not aware that many people with AIDS die of several types of cancer. No one really dies of AIDS—they die of other diseases, having a compromised immune system that can't fight infections.

As I thought about it and unpacked her comment, it occurred to me that Beverly was not saying, "Let's just pretend it's cancer," because she was worried about me or my AIDS diagnosis. No. What Beverly was concerned about in early 1990 was the Spokane Christian community.

Could they survive a couple in leadership who had AIDS? It was actually a good question. People were fearful of AIDS. They were questioning the findings on how the disease was transmitted and were skeptical, especially in conservative rural communities.

But ... this was not cancer. The very statement was an indication of the potential fear, stigma, and discrimination that came packaged with AIDS in 1990 and beyond.

I don't know anyone with cancer who ever spent as much time as we did trying to make people feel comfortable being around us, helping people to not be fearful about my disease, and helping them to feel compassionate to our friends and family who were also infected. I haven't met anyone with cancer who needed to spend time trying to help the medical professionals who were taking care of them feel safe while touching them or drawing their blood. I don't know people with cancer who have been told it is God's judgment that they are sick. Or that they deserved what they got. Or that they were not welcome because of their disease. Or that they needed their own utensils that would be thrown out after every meal. Or that their neighbors were uncomfortable with their children coming to their house. Or that their child was not allowed to go to school.

On the other hand, I've met people with AIDS who have had every single one of these things happen.

As I'm typing this, I almost say, "Let's just pretend it's AIDS, said nobody ever." But then I think of Ebola, leprosy, and the many complicated diseases around the world that also come with fear and stigma. Even lung cancer receives judgment. "Well, they were a smoker." Or diseases associated with obesity. "Well, if they would've just lost that weight, they wouldn't have gotten diabetes" or "had that heart attack." You get the picture.

But, in 1990, in Spokane, AIDS was the disease that carried the most social shaming and fear; no one wanted it to affect their community.

So, Beverly, I'm sorry to say, but this was definitely not cancer.

MARY AND MAGIC

Don't put off your happy life.

Anonymous

In the summer of 1991, our whole family traveled to the Christian youth camp in Canada because Scott was the camp manager for a month. This was the same camp I'd spent spring break at almost a decade before as a college student. The camp is in a remote area of British Columbia surrounded by water and mountains, it is only accessible by boat or seaplane. Because of this, each week two doctors come with their families to volunteer at camp and attend to the medical needs of the three hundred campers and roughly two hundred staff and volunteers residing there.

One week I kept sitting at meals with one of the camp doctors, but for some reason, his wife was never with him. So, I asked him, "Where is your wife, Mary? Is she doing okay? Is everything all right?"

His answer left me dumbfounded: "Well, thank you for asking. Actually, Mary is dealing with a pretty significant illness. You see, six years ago she had a blood transfusion from a postpartum hemorrhage. A couple of years ago she found out that the blood was infected with HIV and now she is very sick with AIDS."

I stared at him in disbelief. It was like hearing my own story repeated back to me. Up to that point, I'd never met another woman with AIDS. I began to tell him our own, very similar, story.

I met Mary that evening in her cabin. Although she had been infected with HIV over a year after I had, her disease was progressive in spite of the best available treatment at the time. Mary was very, very sick.

After camp, I stayed in touch with Mary. She lived north of Seattle and had been a nurse who specialized in programs for children with developmental disabilities. With her husband, she had restored a Victorian mansion, and her face lit up when telling me about her whimsical wallpaper of frogs that danced around the light fixture on the high ceiling in her music room. She had bought a flute, meaning to take lessons in that special room. That was all before HIV set in.

A local newspaper ran an article about the amazing job Mary had done educating her community about AIDS. We talked on the phone a few times after camp; there was no internet at that time, so we also passed a few letters through the mail, the old-fashioned way. I was always amazed at Mary's calm and her wisdom. She talked about her kids and her garden. She was encouraging. I don't think she realized just how special it was for me to meet another mom dealing with HIV.

The fall after I met Mary, another AIDS event happened that rippled through my life in unexpected ways. I'll never forget waking up on November 7, 1991, and turning on the news to find that every station was talking about Magic Johnson having AIDS.

First, I loved the NBA. In our last year of college, my roommate and I had the opportunity to go to several Seattle Sonics games because she was dating one of the players. In 1978 and 1979 the Sonics went to the playoffs, and, for a few of those games, we were courtside.

I also loved Magic Johnson. He's one of my favorite players—so easy to like on and off the court.

That day, watching Magic Johnson's announcement, like most of the world, I was stunned, even shocked. Everyone I knew was, all of a sudden, talking about HIV and AIDS. At that time, most of my acquaintances and many of my friends had no idea that I was infected with HIV.

I know there were people, especially heterosexual people, who were surprised when Rock Hudson died of AIDS in the mid-1980s. But Rock Hudson was my parents' age, so most of my friends didn't really pay much attention. On this day, when Magic Johnson told the world that he had AIDS, the world woke up in a big way to the fact that this was not just a gay disease. It was not a disease that discriminated.

Watching Magic Johnson on television, I thought, "He doesn't even look sick." He was sharing quite a bit about how he felt good, how he was working out a lot, and about how he was expecting to live a long time. In a roundabout way, Magic Johnson's announcement that day, in all of its sadness, gave me hope.

I looked at him, thinking to myself, "This is not a picture of death. This is a seemingly very healthy person."

When everyone started talking about the fear surrounding Magic Johnson passing on this virus by playing basketball, in another strange and unexpected way, this helped me see that all of the things happening to me were also happening to other people. I didn't feel alone anymore.

I admired Magic Johnson's courage to go public right away, to come out and say, "I have AIDS" a few days after he found out. At that point in my life, I didn't have that kind of courage. I admired it, but I didn't want to join in. It would be three more years before we went public with my diagnosis. I've wondered a few times if Magic ever regretted telling his story to the public so fast. My guess is, he was possibly wanting to stay in control of that announcement, because, at some point, the media might have leaked it anyway.

The biggest life change for me from the Magic Johnson announcement, other than feeling hopeful, was that I began to work out, and not in a small way. I joined a gym and signed up for an aerobics class. For most of my life I had been in really good shape. As a kid, I was in ballet for ten years and was a gymnast in junior high and high school. In college, I started running, often spending weekends at local fun runs. As a high school teacher in the early '80s, I was one of the cross-country coaches.

When I started having kids, I kept up a rigorous workout routine. I even ran regularly until I was eight months pregnant with Laura. By the time I reached my third pregnancy in four years and faced the reality of having three small children, it all caught up to me. I stopped working out. I hadn't done any serious exercise since Ryan was born. Even if I had tried, being HIV-positive, I probably wouldn't have had the energy to work out during those years after Ryan was born.

When I walked into the room, it was clear I wasn't just out of shape, I was out of style. If you've ever watched a '90s Jane Fonda workout video, you get the picture. Women with permed hair and full-on made-up faces sporting the brightest combinations of spandex leotards bounced cheerfully like energizer bunnies to eight-count beats of the latest popular songs.

This aerobics class that I showed up for wasn't a beginning class; it wasn't even an intermediate class. No, the class I signed up for, during the only time I had available, was for advanced students. I had no idea what I had signed up for until I was smack dab in the middle of the first session.

I frantically wondered, "What did you get yourself into?"

The pace started at a sprint and then went into hyper speed. I'm amazed I didn't quit the first week. I just kept thinking about Magic Johnson and the fact that he was playing basketball at the level of the NBA, despite being HIV-positive. Surely, I could survive this class.

Eventually, I started feeling stronger, better than I had in a very long time. It also seemed I was getting sick a little less often. The exercise class eventually led to long walks and then short jogs and then, again, I was running!

Running was something that I thought I would never be able to do again, something that HIV had taken from me. I learned an important lesson through this exercise transition. I learned to never again say I couldn't do something because of AIDS. I might say that I couldn't do something, but I would always add, "for now."

I have in the past many years said to friends who are also dealing with major illnesses, "You are only giving that up for now, not necessarily forever."

Mary died in the early fall two years after I met her; she was only forty-four years old. I read about her death when her husband mailed me her obituary.

After Mary died, the local newspaper ran an article about her life. Her pastor told of Mary's desire to live. He talked about how Mary simply just kept choosing to live. Even up until five minutes before she died, she was choosing to live.

That spoke to me. Real courage is choosing to live.

Mary died shortly after I started running again. I don't remember all of the details of her passing, but I do remember what I did afterward. I ran. I ran for miles. It was as if the thought of her, her life, the family she left behind, the talks we were never going to have again, kept me moving. I ran for Mary, but I think more than that, I ran for myself.

She was the first woman I had met with AIDS, and she

was the first woman I knew who had died of AIDS. I'm not sure what I was running away from or running to, but I do remember wondering why Mary had died and why I got to live. This was something I would grapple with again and again, as I watched more people die of AIDS. I promised Mary that I would try my best to live well. My run that day was a tribute to her life, but it was also a tribute to mine, the life I was privileged and grateful to still be living.

THE QUESTION OF
BLAME

You can't change what's done,
You can't go back in time...
You can't try to mend the broken hearts.

Anonymous

Many people have asked me over the years if I was ever angry or blamed the person who donated the infected blood that gave me HIV. Truthfully, I never even thought of this until someone asked me the first time.

My answer came fairly quickly and easily: "You know, I've never even thought of blaming the person who donated blood. They were trying to be a good Samaritan. I'm sure they had no idea that their blood was infected with HIV. Hypothetically, if I had donated blood before 1990, I also wouldn't have had any idea that my blood was infected with HIV. If I had donated blood, my blood could have possibly infected someone else without my knowledge."

After I was diagnosed, I chalked it up to a freak accident that I'd been infected by the blood transfusion, and not very likely. But then, in early 1991, one of my doctors started asking me if I was thinking of filing a lawsuit against the blood bank that infected me.

At the time, I assumed that all blood banks were

humanitarian organizations that would never make a decision that would harm someone's life. I didn't think of them as businesses that were trying to make money to please their investors and their board of directors. So, I started reading and researching to educate myself on the history of HIV in the blood supply.

In January of 1983, when it was established that HIV was passed, not only by sexual contact, but also through the blood, the Centers for Disease Control and National Institutes of Health started researching if there could be a way to monitor blood products. It became apparent that many hemophiliacs were being infected through the blood product used to help clot blood, AHF (antihemophilic factor) or Factor VIII.

One of the suggestions to make the blood supply safer was to create a better screening process for people who were donating blood. The other idea was to do a surrogate test that could be used to screen potential high-risk donors. In this case, that surrogate was to test for hepatitis B. In 1983, through some research, it was suggested that about 88 to 90 percent of HIV-infected blood could have been screened out of the blood supply, in some regions, if that blood had first been tested for hepatitis B. Most blood-product suppliers opted out of that option because it was cost-prohibitive, and they wanted to save money. They were also concerned that screening would scare away donors and imply that the blood was not safe.

Between 1977 and 1985, the time when HIV was being spread but before a diagnostic test was available, an estimated 26 million people in the US received blood transfusions.

By 1990, the blood-selling industry was worth $2.5 billion. That same year, a boy in Arizona was awarded $28.7 million after being infected with HIV through a blood transfusion. This was the largest settlement at the time, with a few others settling in the $12 million range. In almost every lawsuit where a settlement was "won" by the plaintiff, no one was really winning because they almost always lost their loved one to AIDS before the lawsuit was over.

Even though there were some large settlements, most lawsuits during that time favored the defendant, the blood suppliers. In the late 1980s and early 1990s, the court would usually conclude that the blood suppliers, the blood banks, were following the "standard of care" at that time and, thus, were not responsible. That standard of care had been decided at a meeting in January of 1983 by several government organizations, including the NIH and CDC.

People who had been infected through a blood-clotting product, Factor VIII, while being treated for hemophilia, had an especially hard time in court. Because the product containing HIV was produced by four different companies, it was very hard to track which of them had provided the exact Factor VIII that had infected a particular person. Eventually, there were class action or group lawsuits that ended in settlements for HIV-infected hemophiliacs. In my opinion, the settlements were only a fraction of what they deserved. There was clear evidence that these companies knew they had HIV-contaminated products as far back as 1983 but failed to adequately warn hemophiliacs of the risk or pull their infected products from the market.

One day, this doctor shared with Scott and me that he had been in discussions where the risk of infection by blood products and the cost of lawsuits were discussed. Several people in medical risk management felt that it would probably cost less to pay an HIV-infected person later than to pay for screening tests upfront. The blood banks around the country knew that they might have HIV-infected blood products. They also knew that, eventually, someone might become HIV-positive from their blood and that those people might file lawsuits. It was a risk they could decide to take because, at the time, they were following the "standard of care" set by our government agencies.

"You are that person." He looked right at me. "At some point, they made a decision to save money and not screen thoroughly knowing this might happen to someone."

Knowing I was uncomfortable with the whole conversation, he added, "You know, it's not like you're suing the people down the street. You're suing an insurance company that did the math. Probably a giant insurance company that has a big skyscraper in New York City. They somewhat expected this, so don't feel bad."

We decided to at least look into it. Scott and I found two lawyers in Spokane who were willing to take our case, with whom we discussed the pros and cons. We began the process of filing a lawsuit in the winter of 1992. Our lawyers suggested that we take the kids to have a professional photo shoot. This was the beginning of painting a portrait of a darling, white, Christian family with three beautiful children who had been wronged by a blood bank, and now their mom was going to die.

Even as I was participating in this, I was very aware that the justice system works so much better for some people than for many others. If I had been a single mom, if I did not have the means to find lawyers, if I had been infected by a blood transfusion but had what some would call a sketchy life, other risk factors, things they could question ... there would be no lawsuit, there would be no lawyers, and there would be no possibility of getting a settlement.

To make a long story shorter, it was only a few months before we were offered an out-of-court settlement. It wasn't all that much money when you think that the worst outcome from this was that I would die, and the next best outcome was living a little longer but having huge medical bills and not being able to work or have any salary or income. Not to mention the trauma that this inflicted on my family, on my kids, and the stigma and discrimination experienced because of the nature of AIDS in the 1990s.

We had to decide whether or not to take this settlement. Our lawyers sat us down and had a very frank conversation about our options. Option A was that we take the settlement; we then would have money in the bank immediately to live the best life we could and to have the most experiences with our kids before I died. We would get to move on with our lives. With the three-to-five-year survival plan, this seemed like a good option.

Option B, on the other hand, would be that we not take the settlement and we go to court. With this option, we would probably get a significantly larger settlement, like four to five times more money. Our lawyers anticipated any settlement would probably take years. I would probably die before it was over. Also, we could be on the front page of the paper, every detail of our lives exposed. The prosecution would use every angle in court, most likely bringing up that my brother was also infected and somehow insinuating that he infected me, not the blood bank. Anything and everything was possible and could be skewed to make us look bad in order to save the blood bank money.

It was a fairly easy and obvious decision. All of our thoughts were around our kids, and what would cause them the least amount of anguish and pain, and of innocence lost. We decided on Option A.

We decided that although we might be awarded much more money in court, this settlement would allow us to go on with our lives. And that was priceless.

OPTION A

I'm grateful for always this moment, the now,
no matter what form it takes.

Eckhart Tolle

B y the time we received any money it was the summer of
1992, we expected me to die soon, two of my possible
five years were gone, and time continued to tick away.
So we put the money into three different things to provide
memories spent together, memories of me with our kids.

The first thing we decided to do with the money was
travel. And I'm not talking about a European vacation here.
We wanted to travel and create experiences our kids would
remember. So, with kids in mind, we took a couple of trips
to Hawaii and a few trips to Disneyland. We recorded these
trips with a plethora of photos so that even Ryan, who was
very young, could remember these vacations and could see
pictures of himself with a healthy mom who was having fun.

The second thing that we did with our settlement was
to buy a cabin in Northern Idaho on Priest Lake. It was our
financial advisor who suggested this.

He said to us, "I could put your money in the bank, or
I could put it into stocks and bonds, and it would probably
make a good amount of profit for you. Or, you could take
some of this money and buy a cabin on one of the many
lakes around Spokane. You won't end up with as much

profit, financially, but the amount of profit from the family experiences and relationship building that you will get from that cabin might be worth far more value than anything I could do on the stock market."

The third thing we did was finish the basement of our house. When we bought our house, we liked the idea that it had the potential to expand, by building out a basement which was basically just a cement floor and some unfinished walls. That summer, after the settlement, we began a remodel to add a playroom or rec room, an extra bedroom, and a new bathroom. One of the main reasons we wanted to do this was that we had no space for my parents to stay with us, or, to be frank, we had no space for a caregiver to stay with us. I was well aware that we probably would need that space.

I did do one frivolous thing after that lawsuit settlement came in. I went to Nordstrom, and I bought a complete outfit. By "complete outfit," I mean an outfit including a jacket, shoes, a silk blouse, jewelry, a skirt, and coordinating pants in case I didn't want to wear the skirt. It was something that I had never once done in my whole life. I always had nice clothes, but I usually shopped at the bargain stores; we weren't making a killing being in youth ministry. The only time I went shopping for fancy things or whole outfits was in the summer when Scott's mom would take me shopping for my birthday and get me a few outfits that I could wear at camp. This was different. It was kind of like adult shopping. Maybe even rich-adult shopping, although none of the things I bought were designer brands. I didn't ever do that again, but it was very, very fun to do once.

I never once regretted settling our lawsuit for the amount we did in such a timely manner. We did a lot of living in those next few years that could've been tied up in court proceedings.

In the end, I came to realize after the lawsuit that money brought privilege and privilege brought options. Options that many other people I met with HIV and AIDS did not have. I didn't like that at all, but it was the truth.

TRADITIONS

In the end, it's not the years in your life that count.
It's the life in your years.

Abraham Lincoln

Scott's mom, Eleanor, is the queen of Christmas. From the first year we were married, I spent Christmases at Eleanor and Mel's home in Yakima. Eleanor was the type of person who spent the whole year prepping for the holidays, and she was an expert.

One year, Eleanor had *six* different Christmas trees, each perfectly decorated in a different style. That year, her home was featured in Yakima's Christmas Tour of Homes. People bought tickets to walk through her home at Christmastime.

I was thankful to have Eleanor making Christmas so magical, especially those first few years after my diagnosis when I was getting used to my meds and processing so much. But by the fall of 1993, I was ready to take control of what I could and wanted to be intentional with whatever time I had left. I wanted to leave my children with traditions that they could come back to when I was gone.

Scott and I put a lot of thought into the details of our first Christmas at home in Spokane. Going to the Christmas Eve service at our church was important to me; I had always loved singing Christmas hymns by candlelight and wanted to be able to share that with my kids. I never wanted to force my faith on them, but rather offer them opportunities to find comfort in it the same way that I did and leave them with a way to feel connected to me when I was gone.

We planned a salmon dinner, fancy, yet still kid-friendly, for after the church service, and we decided to eat next to the Christmas tree, sitting on pillows on the floor around the coffee table. It seemed like one of those slightly zany childhood memories that might stick with you once your mom was gone.

That year we began what I consider the most significant tradition of the holidays: having each person share the highs and lows of their year. At the time we were looking for ways that the kids could reflect. They were small children who were going to soon be dealing with adult problems. It seemed like something that could be therapeutic for them in the future, to see that we were all experiencing hard things, but that there were also very good things happening.

To lighten up the night, we played a dice game where everyone ended up with a present. Before they went to bed, the kids each opened two presents from under the tree: pajamas and a special ornament.

That first year, I have to admit, I was exhausted. I admired Eleanor more than ever because I learned that organizing a memorable family holiday is practically a part-time job.

At the end of the night, that first Christmas in Spokane, we had a family dance. Yes ... we were and are a little weird. But we had tricked our kids into going to bed an hour earlier than normal by setting every clock in the house ahead an hour, so Scott thought a dance might wear them out. Oh, the things parents do to survive!

PWA

I am not afraid of storms,
for I am learning to sail my ship.

Louisa May Alcott

When we moved to Spokane, I realized that I would need to find a dentist. Oral health was a priority for me. After I quit teaching, I worked for a dentist. I am one of the few people who don't have to lie to their dental hygienists ... I actually floss regularly! I have fancy toothbrushes and am a stickler for having dental check-ups every six months.

I received a list of possible dental offices to contact that had previously accepted new patients who had HIV. As I began calling down the list of potential dental practitioners, I was met with the same response from every receptionist.

"We are not taking any more PWAs."

The first time I wasn't sure what to do or say, so I just said, "Thank you," and hung up.

The next office I called, I asked the person on the other end of the phone, "What exactly is a PWA?"

There was a pause, and then she said, "A PWA is a person with AIDS."

I continued down the list of more than ten dentists and each one had the exact same response. My brother had warned me that finding dental care was one of the hardest things for HIV-positive people, but I hadn't been prepared for the sting of what it felt like to be reduced to an acronym. Eventually, I remembered a dentist practicing in Spokane who was from my hometown. He indirectly knew our family so I decided to call that dentist and see if he would take me as a patient.

Thank God for small hometowns. I called, and his receptionist was his wife, and she knew my family. My older brother had worked for their men's clothing store when he was in college. I am not exaggerating when I say that tears were coming down my cheeks when she said, "Of course we will see you; let's make an appointment and get you in."

This dentist took incredibly good care of me. He never treated me differently than any other patient. I know this is not the story that a lot of my friends with AIDS experienced; many never found consistent and reliable dental care.

One of the surprising things for me after I was diagnosed with HIV was the fear and negative attitude I would receive from the medical community, the very people who were supposed to help me stay well.

When I started to branch out to medical specialists, whom I was being referred to for the side effects of my medications, almost every receptionist would look at my chart as I was checking in, see I had HIV, and then ask for my coupon.

At first, I had no idea what they were talking about so I kind of jokingly asked, "Are you having a sale?"

Nobody found that funny; they just rolled their eyes. "Your medical coupon." The medical staff automatically thought that I was on public assistance and had medical coupons for Medicaid.

A few other things that they would assume: I didn't have a husband, I was an IV drug user, I was seeking painkillers.

When I had a very sore throat, I went to the lab to

get a culture to see if I had strep. When I arrived at my appointment, I immediately noticed that the technician who was helping me was decked out in a mask, plastic gloves, and a gown—and she looked very nervous.

So I asked her, "Would you be more comfortable if I just swabbed my own throat?" I'm not even sure why I offered this.

With a sigh of relief, she replied, "Oh yes, please!"

She then set the swab on the table, so she wouldn't have contact with my hand. I picked it up, swabbed the back of my throat, and then set it back on the table.

I don't know how she thought she was going to get HIV. Was she expecting the virus to jump out of my body and into hers like some sort of demon possession? She was genuinely frightened of me.

When Teresa was in third grade, she had a terrible stomachache and was vomiting. We took her to the emergency room, met with her pediatrician, and he informed us that she had appendicitis and needed surgery.

He then added, "We'll need to do an HIV test on her before we can operate."

Annoyed, I responded, "Is getting an HIV test protocol for all children needing surgery?"

"No, it isn't protocol," he admitted with an embarrassed look. "I just want her tested because you are HIV-positive, just to be sure."

I paused, breathed deeply, and trying to not look angry, I said, "Teresa has been tested for HIV twice, and she is definitely not infected. What do you imagine that I'm doing with her or to her that would infect her since her last HIV test?"

I also reminded him that he usually didn't know if a patient had a blood-borne disease prior to surgery because many infected people didn't know themselves. Here was one patient, my daughter, whom I could assure him did not have HIV.

He had no good response but repeated that a test was required for the surgery to happen.

So, there it was: our own pediatrician, a family friend, was fearful. Teresa had the HIV test, had the surgery, and then we promptly changed our kids' doctor.

During our first few years in Spokane, Dr. C and I became pretty good friends, and, because he had known my sister professionally, one time when she came to town, we all went out for happy hour.

Over a couple of beers that night he said to me, "If you ever need to go to the emergency room, you should call me first."

This made me curious, so I asked him, "Why?"

He went on, "Well, sometimes in the ER, when someone with AIDS comes in, they just give them to the med students to practice on. I don't want anyone practicing on you, so just call me."

This didn't surprise me. I mean, everyone was expecting us to die, so "practicing" medicine on us made complete sense. If someone is going to die anyway, then why not use those people as a teaching tool? Plus, don't kid yourself, those experienced doctors, they didn't want to be anywhere near someone who had HIV. In a way, I respected the med students. When all of the experienced doctors were avoiding us, those doctors in training just did their job.

SADNESS

Sadness is but a wall between two gardens.

Khalil Gibran

t's okay to be sad. Some things are just sad. One time, I watched as a scenario unfolded where a couple I know, young parents, made an extremely hard decision for their child. The best of the options for their daughter was still devastating and very difficult. I listened to their friends, their acquaintances, college classmates, and their church community being very positive and encouraging them. Hardly a sorrowful word was spoken.

All I wanted to say to them was, "It's okay to be sad."

But it seems there's very little space in our culture to allow people to rest in pain and sadness.

I felt that way in the '90s about the church. It seemed like everyone wanted me to move past any sadness as fast as possible. Many people offered miraculous God solutions, as soon as they could think of them. Others reassured me that God was going to use my story in remarkable ways. This did not help.

Sadness is uncomfortable. I think one of the reasons that I settled into depression was that there weren't a lot of spaces to be publicly sad. I stuffed my sadness away; on the outside, I lived my life as positively as I could while on the inside, my spirit was slowly dying. I'm no therapist, but it seems when people skip grieving and aren't honest about loss, their emotions and sadness come out sideways. For me, that sideways grief usually showed up as depression.

On one of those sad days in 1993, alone and dealing with the "three to five," I wrote about it in my journal:

> Deep inside I have had an unending feeling of sadness. I've been infected by a gross and ugly virus I can't get rid of. It feels like I can never be clean again. Something will forever be wrong with me.
>
> This sadness overflows even stronger when I think of my children. I feel like I've messed up their lives and have made it so our whole family cannot be "clean." We are tainted with this disease.
>
> This sadness continues as I think of Scott. This virus has come between Scott and me. It has robbed us of some of our most private intimacy. Sexually, Scott and I can never be as physically close as we used to be. It has literally come between us.
>
> I am sad because I've become more limited in my abilities, and this virus has robbed my future and limited my dreams. I am sad because as much as I learn, as much hope as I can muster, as much "good" that God can make of this, all of that can't make this virus go away. It isn't going away. I am stuck to live with it and to die from it. Deep within me, there is a well of sadness about that. I am

sad, and I am still grieving. I find it difficult to not be in control and to give up more and more control daily.

This is my sadness. This is the heart of my depression. This is the robber of my hope. Cry with me, God. I can do nothing more than be honest about my hurting life. This is my valley and I admit, it is a dark place.

Everyone needs to be able to find a space where they can be honest. Even inappropriately honest—a socially unacceptable kind of honest. For me, this wasn't found very often in the faith community. I found the most freedom with my brother, with his friends, and eventually with some of the women in my Bible study. They allowed me to be pissed, to cry, to cuss, to blame God, to find no lesson learned or happy outcome. I went to several therapists during this time, but none of those compared to these friends. They were my therapy.

ON PREPARING YOUR KIDS FOR YOUR IMPENDING DEATH

A mom's hug lasts a long time after she lets go.

Unknown Author

When we first moved to Spokane I made friends slowly, whereas Scott had a larger group he interacted with at work. What we really lacked and missed were grandparents close enough for our kids to see regularly; our nearest relatives were two hundred miles away. So, Scott and I thought up a plan to remedy this in a small way. You can't truly "replace" people, but the idea was to add to the relational resources available to our children. We wanted to find what we called "special people" for each of them, what some would call "godmothers."

I thought a good fit would be women who were about ten years older than me, who weren't in the middle of mothering small children themselves. The three women I ended up asking I met at our church through Kristine. Over the years, each of them would go above and beyond what I was asking them to do. They all, in their own unique way, would spend quality time with one of my kids, going on "dates," having them as overnight guests, and taking them shopping or to the park. My kids loved being with families who had "big kids," almost like having older cousins who took time to play with them. It felt like a cool thing for a seven- or nine-year-old. Ryan wasn't in school yet when his special person said yes to my request. Her offering to me was time; she would babysit Ryan in the middle of the day—for free!

Truthfully, I hoped that these women would get to know my kids while I was still here, to better offer comfort and support to them when I was gone. What I didn't expect was that all three of these women ended up being substitute moms for me personally. All of them helped me to be able to not only have practical support, but also to be truthful and candid about how hard life sometimes was for me. These women were an exceptional gift to me, a treasure that would never have happened had I not found the courage to ask for help when I needed it.

Besides the special people in my kids' lives, I decided that I should also write some kind of document or journal for my kids to read when they grew up. Like I've said, on the three-to-five-year plan, my kids were going to be very young when I died. I started to realize that they would never actually know the adult me; they would just know the "mom" me. They would remember the things that little kids remember about their mom, like how I cooked good food and tucked them in at night. At least I hoped they'd remember even those little things—would those memories fade too?

I decided to write a series of essays, of sorts, about what happened with the blood transfusion and about a lot of various other things I was thinking and feeling. I would end up writing about my faith, my childhood, my love for their dad, and my love for them. The journal ended up taking about a year to write; it wasn't very long. But, for my children, I was hoping it would endure the test of time and in some way bring understanding and peace once I was gone.

I wanted to leave my kids with something tangible, something they could touch, something that could reach out beyond death and finality. Something that would be theirs alone.

Scott and I made several conscious decisions for our kids who were, in all likelihood, about to face a devastating loss. We decided not to move. We had established a community in our neighborhood and school, and we believed their community needed to be familiar and stable. We decided to spend a significant amount of time with extended family, which meant long drives on the weekends to family birthdays and celebrations, hoping to create a strong identity and a sense of belonging to the greater group of relatives.

Lastly, I tried to take care of myself. Maybe that seems like an obvious thing to do, but with the side effects of my medications and the exhaustion, doing the healthy things took an amazing amount of focus and effort. I wrote about this in my journal in 1994:

> I take care of myself more for my children than for any other reason. When I don't feel like going to the gym to work out, I remind myself that I'm fighting for "days." Every bit of time I can bargain for is one more memory that my kids and I can have together, one more thing I can see them do, one more experience we can share.
>
> I pray for time to see them get bigger, to grow wiser and stronger. I'm fighting for the dream of seeing their first date, their sporting events, their concerts, to see them driving

cars and graduating from high school. There was a time when I wasn't sure if I would see them all graduate from kindergarten. Ryan is finishing kindergarten in a few months, praise God!

So, I continue to look forward to braces, glasses, bras, slumber parties. I look forward to adolescence because to see it for me will be a gift. To fight with a headstrong teenager will be a blessing. I can't wait.

So I try to take care of myself and look to the future in a way that doesn't cause me to miss out on what is happening today. Today was a gift, too, one that I don't want to ignore or take for granted.

THE PRAY-ERS

There are thoughts which are prayers.
There are moments when, whatever the posture
of the body, the soul is on its knees.

Victor Hugo

I prayed for more years, more time. I tried hard to believe all of the Christian positive sayings being thrown my way: When God closes a door, He opens a window. Everything happens for a reason. God doesn't give us more than we can handle. God will work everything for good for those who love Him.

I tried hard to be good enough, worthy enough, and positive enough for these outcomes. Every logical bone in my body, the logic I had always leaned on, reminded me that bad things happen every day to good people. Why would God choose to save some good people and not others? It was very difficult to have something happening to me that had almost no possibility of having a good outcome. To be totally out of control with no sign that it would change.

I decided all the typical positive sayings were ridiculous. What were my kids going to think of God if we said these things to them and then I died? That God didn't love us? That we weren't good enough?

These "quotes" made me feel like somehow if I didn't get healthier my demise would be my own fault.

Christian clichés. Did anyone ever tell me those were stupid at the time? I was not a Biblical scholar, but I knew enough about the Bible to know that none of these sayings were in it, at least not in the context in which they were being doled out.

I was, however, a believer in miracles. I was a believer in miracles for *other* people.

One day I got a call from a friend, Scott's boss's wife. She asked me what she could pray for. She said that she and two other women were meeting once a week to pray for me. That was the sole purpose for which they were getting together, and she would need me to share prayer requests.

So, every week she would call, and I would tell her things to pray for. The interesting thing was, I never once asked to be healed of HIV. I didn't ask because I never believed that was a prayer that would ever be answered.

To put this in perspective, I processed almost everything first, and sometimes solely, through my head. I am a high thinker, low feeler. While sharing these prayer requests my brain kept wondering, "Why on earth, with all of the suffering, poverty, and injustice ... why would God choose me to be the one to heal from HIV?" I just did not think that the God of the universe would pick a privileged, upper-middle-class, white woman who already believed in Him to be the first person to be cured of AIDS.

So, I didn't ask for that prayer.

JOYCE

Larger-than-life characters make up
about .01 percent of the population.

Tom Hanks

There have been a few silver linings woven into my AIDS story, and one of those was my friendship with Joyce Claypool. I am almost certain our relationship would not have happened any other way. I could write a whole other book about Joyce Claypool; she was larger than life itself.

On August 29, 1993, I opened the local newspaper, the *Spokesman Review*, and there on the front page sat an article about a little girl named Kara Claypool, a beautiful five-year-old, who was announcing that she was starting kindergarten in the fall at one of Spokane's public schools, and she was showing up with "full-blown AIDS."

Her mother, Joyce Claypool, who was interviewed for the article, believed strongly in education and was determined to enlighten her community to the fact that Kara could come to school and not be a threat to any other child. In truth, the other kindergarten students, with their runny noses and their uncovered coughs, were a way bigger danger to Kara's health.

This was big news in Spokane. Although there had been other HIV-positive students in the district, they had chosen to remain anonymous.

The article said, "5-year-old Kara may be taking an unprecedented leap into honesty about AIDS when she enters Willard Elementary on Thursday."

Announcing their plan regarding the situation, the school district said that there would be a meeting for all of the parents at Willard Elementary School who had children in Kara's class, and one later for the rest of the parents in their community. The district would educate parents on the facts about AIDS and give them the opportunity to meet Kara's mom, Joyce, to hear her personal story and ask her questions.

The article explained that Kara had been born HIV-positive and then developed an AIDS diagnosis soon after. Joyce told the newspaper that she had passed the virus to Kara after she had been infected by her husband, who was an intravenous drug user. Kara's dad died in 1990. Joyce went on to explain that her two older sons were not infected.

My favorite part of the school district's response was that they said it was okay if parents didn't want their child in Kara's classroom, but their child would have to change schools and go to kindergarten elsewhere. The school district decided to implement this policy because they believed that Kara posed no harm to any other student. BAM! I was delighted to see how well the Spokane School District handled the whole situation.

Spokane was and is a conservative, very "red," kind of town. I was so happy that reason and facts prevailed. Only one family chose to remove their child from Kara's class. Both the Willard Elementary principal and the parents who were interviewed for the article later said that they received multiple calls and letters from anonymous people telling them to reverse their decision.

Joyce stated in the article, "I believe in being totally and brutally honest about this whole thing."

This was one of many times that Joyce Claypool would publicly use her family and her influence to make life a little easier for many others dealing with HIV and AIDS, including my family. Our instinct as parents, often, is to protect our children. It took a special kind of courage to choose what was best for the community at large, potentially over what was easiest for her own child.

Dr. Allen Crocker, a pediatric AIDS expert studying schools and infected children, was quoted in the article, saying about Kara, "One part of me says she's at the front edge of our culture and I'm proud of her and her mother. Another part of me says she's going to get hurt."

When I first read the article about Joyce, I was not only impressed with this family but also excited to meet this woman who was in my city, a woman dealing with AIDS who had kids! From the article I immediately saw that Kara and Ryan were the same age; I also assessed that her two boys had to be about the same age as my girls. I made an appointment to visit the Spokane AIDS Network. Joyce had mentioned in the article that she had been a speaker with this organization. So, I was pretty sure they would know how to find her. I went to the SAN office, and I asked to have a meeting with a case manager. I started out by telling my own story and then I said I'd seen the article about Joyce Claypool and that her kids were the same age as mine. I was wondering how I could meet her.

She smiled kindly, then said, "I just don't think Joyce is in a space to meet new people right now."

That was it. I didn't know how to respond. I left the office disappointed.

A year and a half later, in the spring of 1994, I went to a meeting for women infected and affected by HIV. That night I met two other women who were HIV-positive, Joyce and Camie.

When I introduced myself to Joyce and told her that I was HIV-positive, the first thing she said to me was, "Well, where have you been?"

I told her I'd tried to meet her a couple of years earlier but was told she wasn't in a space to meet me. "Whaaaat?" she said, in total disbelief.

Joyce and I were both sad and a little pissed off. To think that both myself and this woman, whom I grew to love dearly, missed a couple of years of friendship because someone else decided what we needed. It made both of us angry, and for good reason.

Now that she was in my life, we made up for lost time. Joyce had a faith in God that I deeply admired. Despite some shitty life circumstances, she wasn't mad at God, and often had a more positive outlook than I did. As much as I could talk to others about having HIV, what it was like to live with it and prepare to possibly die of AIDS, it was a true gift to be with Joyce and not have to explain the hard feelings because she understood on a deeper, unspoken level. Especially on the "mom" level where we both feared not being there to see our kids grow up. We were truly kindred spirits. Thankfully, our kids hit it off, as well, and my kids began asking to come along to meetings so they could play with the Claypool kids.

Joyce's complete openness and bravery in sharing her whole story, regardless of the judgment she received from some, made me feel that I too could be public about my HIV diagnosis and also use my story to dispel stigma and educate others.

TELLING PEOPLE

It happened again today. I am just now becoming acquainted with a woman whose son is one of Ryan's friends. I see her every week at my Bible study, several times a week at his preschool, and one other time at church on Sunday morning. I have been slowly getting to know her for the last six months and it's been great until today.

Today is the day when all of my trivia ran out. She knows all of the interesting, and uninteresting, regular things about me and my family. Today's the day when everything in the deep part of me was aching to be known. I just got to the end of the insignificant and had to stop because the inner me said it's too risky, too costly, and too scary. I had to stop and hope she has the wisdom to know that there is much more inside.

It's just from here it will be slow. It will take time, trust, and timing. It always comes to this now with people. There were days when I used to lay out my life to people right off.

I really had very little to hide. Those days ended with AIDS.

I try not to second-guess how people will respond to the rest of me. I pray they will have the maturity and the strength to handle all of this mess, but I know most of the education and understanding will have to come from me.

So, I wait. I wait until I have the strength to walk another person through this chaos. Until then, I remain unknown.

Julie's Journal, 1994

So ... what exactly did telling someone I had HIV entail? It usually started by initiating a coffee date; after all, it was the '90s, and like the characters on *Friends*, our lives played out over vanilla lattes. My kids still didn't know my diagnosis, so this wasn't a conversation I could have at home. After securing a private corner table and nervously talking about trivial things, I'd just launch into my story. Once I finished, I'd sit there, staring at my poppyseed muffin in the inevitable awkward silence punctuated by the steaming whistle of the barista frothing milk, patiently waiting to see how they'd take it.

People reacted in all kinds of ways. Some knew a lot about HIV, making it easier. Other times I would spend a good amount of time dispelling misinformation, which often would include an explanation that it was astronomically improbable to get AIDS from a toilet seat.

I calmed fears and occasionally had to help someone stop crying because they became emotional ... about my disease. Even though I was the sick person, it fell to me to be a calm voice of reason, an educator, even adding humor to ease the sense of complete discomfort many people revealed.

These coffee dates could go on for hours. I wanted to be sure to answer every question, making sure no one was left with any reason to be afraid of me or my family.

It was exhausting. If I did this once or twice that would be one thing, but this was how I told people those first four years. Anytime I wanted a real friend in a meaningful relationship, when I wanted any kind of emotional intimacy or support, I needed to go down this road.

I was extra nervous when I decided to tell my neighbor, Paula. Giving this kind of personal information to a neighbor was risky. Once again, I remembered reading about the Ray family in Florida, whose neighbors burned down their house to keep them from putting their HIV-infected children in the local school. I wasn't at all expecting this reaction from Paula, but I didn't know who she would tell and where it would go.

Also, I counted on Paula; she was already a key person in my support system. Her son was Laura's best friend, and we traded babysitting each other's kids because they were in half-day kindergarten. There were all kinds of ways this could go poorly.

In the end, Paula had one of the most chill responses of anyone I ever told. As a nurse, she relied on facts and already had a lot of accurate information about HIV. When I told her, she began to ask if I needed anything more from her. Unlike most of my one-on-ones, Paula flipped the whole conversation to be about me, how she could be a better friend and support me. This was different and new and, as you can imagine, led to one of the most meaningful friendships I had in Spokane. When Paula left my house that day, I breathed a big sigh of relief.

As it became clear that we would soon be telling our kids,

I felt an urgency to talk to anyone we knew who would be offended if they heard about it secondhand.

I looked forward to someday not having to do this anymore. I was ready for everyone to just know so I could get on with my life. I wanted people to get past my diagnosis and begin to see me as a regular person who just happened to be managing a disease.

CAREGIVING

It's all very well to read about sorrows
and imagine yourself living through them heroically,
but it's not so nice when you really come to have them,
is it?

L.M. Montgomery, Anne of Green Gables

As more and more people came to know about my disease, something happened that surprised me. Even though my HIV status was more open, I continued to lie, a lot. What I didn't anticipate was that every person who knew was now going to ask me how I felt, and how I was doing, every time I ran into them.

I never felt great. Side effects from the HIV medications alone challenged me daily. The worst was nausea, constantly balancing what was in my stomach to keep from vomiting. Timing was everything, and an empty stomach became my worst enemy. Fatigue loomed as another challenge, and managing three small children left me dragging. Life became a minute-by-minute drain, and, let's just say, there was never enough coffee. Other side effects varied, everything from numbness in my hands and feet to dizziness and yeast infections everywhere, but especially in my throat.

Telling the truth to every person who asked was depressing. Every. Single. Time.

I would receive their sympathy, which would be long and

drawn out, constantly reminding me that I didn't feel great. Inevitably, people would avoid me because who wants to keep having that conversation? I felt that telling the complete truth would be ridiculous. I began to form an inner circle of people whom I chose to be completely honest with. Not everyone could handle my true life, and I didn't judge them for that; I totally understood. I tried to choose my people wisely.

To everybody else who asked how I was doing, I would just say, "I'm doing great." Or if I was sick, I mean, really sick, I would say, "I'm struggling a little but doing okay," and try to leave it at that.

But the one person who always had the complete picture of what was going on with my disease was Scott.

There are so many layers to a relationship, especially a long marriage, when one person becomes the caregiver of the other. I am sure that books have been written about this and I probably should've read one of them by now, but I haven't. I've simply lived it.

Scott, like many spouses whose partner is sick, constantly stepped up, performing many of the things I'd done, but often was too sick to do. After a full day at work, he'd come home, make dinner, give the kids their baths, prepare their lunches for the next day at school, and on and on.

As I watched all of this from my bed or the couch, knowing I couldn't help, guilt, depression, and humiliation would threaten to consume me. I could do very little to share the load. Being forced out of my role as caregiver and homemaker felt frustrating, like I'd lost a part of myself. Being sidelined made me sad, and often my emotions came out sideways as irritation or anger. Ironically, the person who absorbed these moods was Scott, who was doing his best to be positive and keep the family going.

Add to that stress the possibility that my HIV could be passed to him. The layers of complication and worry were unending.

That's a little snapshot of what Scott dealt with, the whole time showing up to work at a youth ministry organization where being a positive leader and role model was his job, a job we needed, not only for the income but especially for the health insurance. In the early 1990s, once you had a major illness you could be denied coverage from all other insurance companies for that pre-existing condition. No company wanted to take on AIDS. So basically, it was a good thing Scott liked his job and did it well because there was no option to change jobs if we wanted to have health insurance.

On one occasion when Scott and I had gone up to Priest Lake for a romantic time away, the trip culminated with me throwing up my drugs and camping on the bathroom floor.

I looked at Scott from my spot next to the toilet, tears filling my eyes, and I asked, "I'm a good person, aren't I? I mean, am I?"

He assured me I was.

"Then why did this happen?" I asked.

Scott not only had to carry the logistical burdens, but he also had to handle the unending stream of unanswerable questions. Scott had to have questions of his own, but he never added them to my long list. He had to stuff a ton of his own feelings so our family could survive, so he could be the one holding it together the best he could while I was falling apart physically and mentally.

I think the caregiver role is often the most exhausting, the most under-appreciated, and the most difficult because hardly anyone asks about the caregiver.

And for Scott Lewis, even if they did ask how he was doing, he would not tell them the truth. If Scott admitted that he was not doing well, that would feel, to him, like one more problem to be admitted to a sea of problems that already existed. It would also feel, to my husband, like somehow he was failing at his caregiver job.

DUNCAN GARDENS

To the world, you might be one person,
but to one person, you may be the world.

Unknown Author

One day in my bedroom, trying to match my favorite denim skirt with coordinating earrings, Teresa sat watching me on my unmade bed. I loved these moments, chatting with her in the short time between waking and flying out the door.

Then, casually, Teresa asked, "How did your friend Mary die of AIDS?"

Trying not to look alarmed and wondering how this question suddenly came out of thin air, I remembered she had just started AIDS education at school, often saved for the end of the school year.

I calmly replied, "Mary had a blood transfusion before the blood bank started testing their blood for HIV."

Teresa got this god-awful look on her face, "Mom! You had a blood transfusion! Could you have AIDS?"

My heart sank.

"Well, I could have AIDS."

Teresa looked at me and asked the question I had dreaded and feared ever since that August day four years earlier, "Do you? Do you have AIDS?"

I was not ready for this question. Nothing in me was going to answer this question truthfully.

I looked at her and without hesitation replied, "No, I don't have AIDS."

Technically, I only had an HIV-positive diagnosis at that time. But the writing was on the wall: I couldn't lie forever; one of my children was asking. The worst thing would be for her to find out from someone else, to learn that her mom was lying to her.

Needing to tell the kids was fast approaching. This is what I wrote in my journal that day in 1994:

> Several of the questions people ask me concerning being HIV-positive revolve around my children. They ask things like ... What about your kids? ... How does it feel to think about your kids growing up without a mother? ... How do you function knowing the pain your children may someday have to bear? ... How do you prepare your kids for a disease like AIDS?
>
> The questions go on and on.
>
> To tell the truth, I hate these questions. I hate them because they are hard, and so far, I've found no guidebook or manual with advice on how to tell your children you may die soon. I haven't thought of a clear-cut way to communicate that they may be in for a life of pain and separation. It's a very hard situation, and I'm not sure there are any right ways or wrong ways to go about it.
>
> Thinking about the pain my children will probably have to go through, the loss they

will feel, the loneliness they will endure ... sometimes it's more than I can bear, and I become overwhelmingly sad for them. I have never lost a close family member. Both my parents and all three of my siblings, their spouses, and their children are alive. My own children will have to experience a loss far greater than I have had in my life. Wow ... I have no idea how to prepare them for that; I feel inadequate and helpless.

All I can say is I hope and trust that God will use this bad situation to make them strong, compassionate, and loving people. But that all seems so far off. Right now, the reality is that telling our kids will be the hardest thing I've ever had to do.

This is adulthood at its worst.

When we moved to Spokane, the week after I found out I was HIV-positive, I was absolutely certain that my kids were way too young to handle the news that I was infected with the virus that caused AIDS, that I was probably going to die young. At the time they were two, four, and six years old. And now my ten-year-old was asking me if I had AIDS. It was obvious we needed to tell our kids. We debated for a while about just telling Teresa, but after living for four years faking it, hiding it, and lying about it, I felt like that was too much of a burden for a ten-year-old. So we decided to tell all three kids. The heart-wrenching thing was that Ryan was only six. Six years old. The age that I had said, four years earlier, was way too young to tell Teresa.

The first thing we did to prepare was visit a child psychologist, a counselor, to get advice about how to present this information. The counselor, a middle-aged woman who specialized in childhood grief and loss, very calmly asked us about our situation and wondered out loud, "What were our biggest questions?" We told her our story and that we were seeking advice or suggestions regarding telling our children about my disease.

She responded with this: "Well, for a child, the very worst thing they fear would be to lose their mother."

I stopped listening after that. We left, and I just kept thinking, "Thanks for that."

Her words made me feel like whatever we said to our kids was going to be devastating. I didn't want to crush their spirits. I didn't want to take away their innocent joy. I certainly didn't want to put a heavy burden of fear and worrying upon them. For me, this appointment with the child counselor was not helpful. It increased my worry and anxiety and gave me a knot in my stomach every time I thought about how and when we would do this.

I have a difficult time in emotional or sad conversations. I often get teary-eyed and choked up; I'm one of those people who even cries when I see a sappy commercial on TV. Scott, on the other hand, is almost always calm and steady. Because of this, both of us decided it might be best if Scott told the kids and then I answered their questions later. Part of me felt cowardly that I couldn't do this myself, but being overly emotional might increase their worry and concern and make them more fearful.

We also decided that, because our kids were at such different ages developmentally and had varying amounts of knowledge about HIV, he would tell them one at a time. We thought sharing the news individually but at the same location would make part of their experience similar, something they could share.

Scott wanted to find a place to tell them that would be special and private, a place with few interruptions or distractions for the kids—a sanctuary of sorts that would allow for whatever emotions might come out. He scouted around for a couple of days and decided on Duncan Gardens, a beautiful English garden in Spokane's Manito Park. In the middle of the garden was a large fountain with steps around it. This spot was where Scott decided to tell them about my diagnosis, a calm and beautiful oasis surrounded by flowers, a memorable place that the kids could come back to if they wanted.

On Friday, June 17, 1994, starting at ten in the morning, Scott told our children one by one that their mom had a fatal disease. Teresa knew quite a bit about HIV because she was older and had learned a lot in school. Laura knew less. Ryan knew nothing, so Scott told Ryan by comparing the effects of HIV on the body to a video game.

He told each one that this was not secret information, but it was private and personal. It was their own information to share with whomever they wanted in whatever way they wanted. Their dad also reassured them that we were okay, that my doctors knew what they were doing, and that they didn't need to worry.

When they got home, I asked each child if they had any questions; there weren't many. I think processing the information was overwhelming. The next day, again, I asked Laura if she had any questions. All she said was, "This isn't going to happen. I'm not going to think about it anymore."

The last thing planned that day, after the gardens, was to do something fun. The week was the opening of the Disney movie *The Lion King* and we decided to go as a family to ease all of the seriousness and tension from the day. We didn't know anything about *The Lion King* when we decided this.

One of the long-standing jokes in our family is that it is probably not a good idea to tell your kids that one of their parents might die and then take them to a movie where, in the first half hour, one of the parents of the main character dies.

The kids later laughed at us, "Yah, way to go, telling us Mom is going to die and then taking us to see Mufasa trampled by hyenas and poor Simba on his own."

Parent fail for sure!

In hindsight, it's a Disney animated movie—of course we should have expected it to start out with one of the parents dying. That's the Disney formula!

At the time, in the theater, Scott and I just looked at each other and were dying a little inside. For all of our careful planning and efforts to control the situation, this was the one thing we had overlooked. Neither of us thought to find out what the movie was about. It's one of the only things the kids remembered about the whole day.

The last part of our plan, to help the kids process all of this new and serious information about their mom, was to take them to a safe place apart from school friends and the greater community. So, the next day we left for British Columbia to spend a month back at camp. Scott was set to be the camp manager, and we had arranged for several close friends and my parents to join us during that time. This was an attempt to have as much control as possible in a situation that wasn't controllable.

As it had been for Scott and me in the past, this beautiful spot in the middle of nature was once again a place of refuge—this time for our children. It was the perfect place for all of us to process a life of being public with the fact that our family was living with AIDS. We felt a ton of support from the staff. Most were people we'd known for years who already knew about my diagnosis. One woman just happened to be a grade school counselor. She intentionally looked for opportunities to have one-on-one time with each of the kids and asked questions to help them express how they were feeling about my diagnosis.

But mostly, we just enjoyed being together in this idyllic place. The camp looks like a giant treehouse built on a rock in the middle of nowhere, surrounded by mountains running directly down into the water, tucked away from the world. Just as we had in previous summers, my kids got to be kids for a month of boating, swimming, singing, and playing, and they got to see me be their regular, normal mom.

ALBERTSONS

Freedom is the only worthy goal in life.
It is won by disregarding things that lie
beyond our control.

Epictetus

After we got home from camp, our lives felt like not a lot had changed. The kids seemed to be doing okay, my HIV status was largely still private, and we were preparing to go back to school. Then, one day in late summer, I was with Ryan at Albertsons buying groceries.

When we got to the checkout, he looked at me, pointed to the checker, and asked, "Does she know you have AIDS?"

It took me a second, but I responded, "Well, she does now."

The woman checking our groceries gave me a nervous smile and proceeded to keep her head down while completing the transaction.

Nothing had changed, but everything had changed. The thought, the idea, that we could in any way control who knew about our family situation was dispelled instantly when we told a six-year-old I had AIDS.

On some level, it was kind of refreshing to just let it be out there. The only way forward was to let go and let it happen. We'd told Ryan that my HIV was his information to share, and to make it otherwise for him would've made it feel like a secret and that he had done something wrong. This was his information, and he was trying to figure out how to put it out into the world. Thus began the new reality in our lives that we were going public with my HIV diagnosis.

A few days after school started that fall, I got a call from Ryan's teacher and she started by saying, "Ryan shared some very interesting information with the class today."

I kind of knew what was coming, "Oh really ... What did he share?"

"Well, we were talking about Africa in class, and he raised his hand and said there was a lot of AIDS in Africa. I told him that was true. Then he went on to tell the class that his mom has AIDS."

She started to apologize to me because she knew this was private information, but I stopped her.

"Well, what he said was true, and it's okay with me if Ryan shares it," I said.

That was that. All of the scary things I thought might happen didn't. No parents called, the teacher did not freak out, the students continued their day, life went on.

I had to believe that part of their reaction was due to another first grader, who was in a different class on the other side of town. Kara, and her mom, Joyce, had spent the past year educating our whole city and school district about families and kids living with and around HIV. I could see clearly, in that moment, that they were a true gift to my children and our family as we began to navigate this public life with AIDS.

I was happy that my HIV was no longer a secret, and that our family could be honest and open. In the fall of 1994, I joined a speakers' bureau with about fifteen HIV-positive people and began a nine-year journey of public speaking about AIDS. My life was changing rapidly, and I had no idea what lay ahead.

I'd lived the last four years orchestrating and controlling everything I could surrounding my disease, but those were behind me. As I looked forward, I was excited and also a little nervous.

I began to realize one new truth: in going public, we were deep in the land of no control.

PART 2

UNLIKELY PARTNERS

HIV SPEAKERS' BUREAU

Out of suffering have emerged the strongest souls;
the most massive characters are seared with scars.

Khalil Gibran

The first time I started to think about the importance of HIV education was not long after I was diagnosed. In October, that first fall in Spokane, when we finally got to move into our new house, Scott's office assistant came by to help us clean after we'd made a mess arranging all of our knickknacks and figuring out the best place to put all of our furniture. She was scrubbing our master bath and then began to clean our toilet and stopped. I could tell something was wrong and she confessed that she felt uncomfortable because she still wasn't sure how HIV was contracted. That was hard to hear, and I did my best to calm her fears and get her as much "protective" gear as we had available to make her feel more at ease.

I mention this because I really admired and respected her that day for being honest and for voicing her fears. That's one thing I would come to learn; most people with fears wouldn't say anything, they would just conveniently stop coming by. They wouldn't actually tell me. This was difficult because I lost the opportunity to discuss their fears and to educate them about my disease.

In this case, on that day in my bathroom, education was

more than a lesson in health. It was about fear, justice, and relationships.

I thought deeply about the value of accurate factual information and the need for HIV education and educators when Dr. Winters gave his fear-based rant at Teresa's grade school, when I watched the world react to Magic Johnson, and when I had coffee date after coffee date telling my friends of my diagnosis during our "closet" years.

And now that we were telling people and were entering a different season of being more public about our lives with AIDS, I had a deep desire to do more to help people understand HIV. I'd always been a big believer in personal stories to change attitudes and prejudice. For four years I had watched my own story change people's views, not only about AIDS in general, but also about the notion that some people deserved to be infected as a divine judgment.

HIV was barely visible in pop culture in 1994. Chad Lowe had just played an HIV-positive high school student on *Life Goes On* for two seasons and MTV made waves by casting Pedro, an HIV-positive gay man, on *The Real World*, both of which reached only limited audiences. The movie, *Philadelphia*, made the biggest splash culturally. The Oscars that year were filled with celebrities donning red ribbons when Tom Hanks won Best Actor for his portrayal of Andrew Beckett, an HIV-positive man. But Spokane never prided itself on being at the forefront of change. I was reminded daily of the conservative, judgmental attitudes people could have when they began remarking about Hollywood's attempt to include AIDS on television and in films.

I first heard about the Spokane HIV/AIDS Speakers' Bureau from Joyce, who had taken me to a couple of presentations. When the coordinators for the speakers' bureau contacted me about joining, I jumped at the opportunity, not only to have something positive to do but also to join a community of people dealing with similar issues as me.

I come from a family that has always placed a high value on education. When I was born, my father was a high school principal and coached football and basketball in a small town where everything entertaining revolved around the local schools, particularly the high school. Eventually, Dad became a school administrator, a superintendent of schools, and my mom became a grade school secretary.

After college I became a high school science teacher because I love facts, I love sharing, and I have always believed that education is power. When I married Scott and began raising a family, I was no longer in a typical classroom, but I continued to teach in other ways. I began to write a curriculum to train youth leaders.

From the beginning of my diagnosis, I could see how much education could change attitudes and break down barriers, fears, and stigma. Joining the HIV/AIDS speakers' bureau was the next logical step.

Tracy and Julie Z, the Spokane HIV/AIDS Speakers' Bureau coordinators, first met me at a cute bistro in Browne's Addition, the oldest neighborhood in Spokane, filled with beautiful Victorian homes and quaint eateries. We sat on their patio in early September of 1994, and over coffee and sandwiches, they explained to me the ins and outs of the speakers' bureau. They presented me with a booklet explaining speaker protocol, facts about HIV, and helpful things to include in my presentations. Tracy admitted that much of the "training" was more likely going to involve observing other speakers and gleaning what resonated with audiences, which largely meant just listening to the questions people asked.

The Spokane speakers' bureau was a joint effort between

the Spokane Regional Health District, a Washington State-run agency, and a local nonprofit, the Spokane AIDS Network. They worked in collaboration on several HIV services to increase their community outreach so as not to compete as providers. Once-a-month speakers' bureau meetings were often held at one of these agencies, although every now and then we met at a home or even in a church basement.

I immediately liked both Julie Z and Tracy and grew over the years to love them. They weren't infected with the virus but were dedicating their lives and careers to helping people, like me, have a better life. They became true advocates, soldiers really, for a disease that desperately needed justice and support.

The Spokane speakers' bureau was a huge transition in my life with HIV. Being a public speaker in my community definitely had pros and cons.

Obviously, I gave up privacy. Going public, I gave up the right to be anonymous. There were many good reasons not to disclose my HIV status, but in becoming a public speaker for a large area of Washington State and Northern Idaho, I gave up that right to privacy. I gave up the right or the ability to control who knew, who I wanted to know, or when I wanted to tell them. Being a complete control freak, this was probably the hardest part for me.

I'd never considered the media. Never thought about reporters and what they might say or print. What it would feel like to be misquoted, and misquoted over and over again. How it might affect my marriage to talk publicly about a sexually transmitted disease ... in schools ... even my own kids' schools. How my relatives would be affected when a talk I gave at a high school in a small rural Eastern Washington town would end up on the front page of their local paper, before they'd shared that information with any of their friends or colleagues.

I knew I was giving up control and privacy, but, really, I had no idea the extent. I learned to use phrases like "off the record," and to begin by asking if there were reporters in the room, and, if so, could they please introduce themselves, and then telling them I did not allow videotaping of my talks. Thank God there were no smartphones or social media yet.

What I gained was the opportunity to educate and a platform to do it. I learned that I was pretty good at public speaking, and not only did that give some value to my situation but also hope to our speakers' bureau that we were actually saving lives. We were trying to keep people from dealing with what we were experiencing by not only sharing our stories but also by educating how to prevent HIV infection in the first place.

This group of advocates was standing together as a united force promoting justice for people who were infected with HIV. One of the biggest things it provided me was community. A community that supported me and understood the things I was going through. A community that saw and experienced the same injustices and stigma I had witnessed and was courageously doing something about it.

Not long after I joined the speakers' bureau, we made a pact, an agreement as a group. We agreed that when we were speaking, people could ask us any question, except one. The one question the audience could not ask us was how we'd gotten infected. We collectively made that decision because it became clear from the questions we were receiving that it was what everyone wanted to know immediately; it was usually the first question asked if a speaker hadn't included it in their presentation. We noticed many people in the audience used this information to form judgments. There was a visible difference both in the amount of empathy and concern being offered infected individuals and in the number of questions being asked of them, depending on how they had acquired the virus.

There were innocent victims, and then there were people who were infected by making what some considered socially unacceptable lifestyle choices, like being gay or using drugs. We called this the "compassion gradient," and we all hated it. That whole scenario was an injustice we thought we could change. We began every presentation from then on saying that we would take all questions except one. If a speaker didn't want to share how they were infected, they had that right and could not be asked. Then we followed that with, "Every one of us is innocent. Nobody deserves this disease. Every person deserves your compassion."

I have to stop and admit, I was uncomfortable when they first decided to not say how we were infected. The thought of people wondering if I'd used injectable drugs or if I'd had an affair with an infected person, since Scott was not infected, bothered me. At the time I lived my life so close to the church at large and even closer to the Christian ministry community in our town. I didn't want people to think poorly of our family or of me. I didn't want to be judged. I didn't even want to be "wondered" about.

But the more I listened to the questions that audiences asked around this topic of modes of infection and saw the subtle and overt judgment attached to those questions, the more my attitude changed; I just wanted to be part of the greater support and advocacy on behalf of all infected people.

I also realized that in trying to change someone's attitude or judgment, there was nothing that compared to a personal relationship, or a personal story told from the heart. As I heard my fellow speakers' bureau members tell their stories and as I digested their wide array of experiences, I grew to love each of them. The need for protecting my image melted away.

It was the first of many things I would learn from the speakers' bureau.

In that first year, while learning about HIV and communicating to different audiences, I would often be on panels with multiple speakers allowing me to hear other people's stories and to see how they presented to a group. A few of the people had been speaking for a long time and knew just when to be serious and when to add in a little humor.

All of the speakers had unique stories, resonating with different people in the audience.

As one fellow speaker, Mark, would put it, "So my personal thing is I don't care what people think about me. You can put it in your head how you want to, or you can discard it. I know for a fact that when I go out and talk there is at least one person listening. I get it all the time. This guy runs up to me in downtown Spokane ... 'AIDS guy, AIDS guy! Hi, you know I remember what you said ... cover your stuff before you hump.' And I'm like, 'Yes! There you go, don't you feel better about yourself?'"

Obviously, my speaking and my story would probably not resonate the same with that young person. But, nonetheless, every one of our stories found a landing place, a soul who could relate. Our differences were our strengths as a whole.

Almost all of us shared our life before diagnosis when we spoke, the years of "not knowing." Those stories also varied, but I think they spoke the loudest to our listeners because people would come with a preconceived idea that if they had HIV, surely they would know it.

"I thought I was quite selective," Mark shared. "I knew who the people were whom I was going home with because they were people I had been going home with for years. I didn't stop and think about who they might be sleeping with when they aren't sleeping with me. And that's the way it goes.

Hardcore realities. Unfortunately, they never sink into you until it's too late."

The sad thing was that many groups, including schools, would try to "special order" a speaker, kind of like selecting something to eat from a menu.

They would say to Tracy or Julie Z, "We are a conservative community so it would be best to send a straight person to talk. We heard about that little girl, Kara, and her mom ..."

Or they'd say, "We really just want positive stories. We don't want to hear about abuse or addiction."

Mark went on to talk about how this felt. "I go to high schools and a lot of schools don't want to hear about my being gay or that I'm an ex-junkie and an alcoholic. I go somewhere else, and they don't want to hear about your abusive family life ... they don't want to hear ... well, everybody has something they don't want to hear."

He went on, "I went to Gonzaga last time and this girl wrote down in her evaluation that she didn't care about my language. I wish I knew who she was because I would walk up to her and say, 'God damn it, you.' Because a lot of people on the speakers' bureau would like to say it's really nice to get up here and say, well, gosh darn it, we have AIDS and we're really fucking pissed. It's not a fun disease."

The truth was, people could just be cold and uncaring. After sharing the most intimate details of your life and the fact that you, like many of your friends, would possibly die soon ... well, sometimes speaking sucked, and it sucked more often for some people than for others.

So, often as a group, we turned to humor to cheer us all up, and believe me, most of our humor was dark and twisted. At first, humor seemed inappropriate, but, as I got to know these fellow speakers who were living with HIV, I saw that humor was a key survival skill.

We'd be sitting at a meeting and two people would be sharing a coke and someone would say, "Oh, you don't have AIDS, do you?"

Then one would shriek, "My God, did you hear what that guy just asked that other man?" The chant would go out, "Drink it, drink it!" And we would all laugh out loud.

We laughed because we were exhausted from constantly trying to convince people that they couldn't "get AIDS" from sharing utensils or food. There were speakers in the room whose own families had made them use paper plates and disposable silverware, being afraid that washing the regular dishes would not kill the virus. That was heartbreaking to imagine, so we just made it into our own joke and laughed, because, well, we were tired of crying.

We made fun of fear, we made fun of pills, we made fun of getting skinny, and we pretty much made fun of death and dying. We were sick, and so was our humor.

Humor was also key in giving presentations. If you happened to be talking about how HIV-positive people were being treated poorly, or how naïve, unaware, or callous people could be, the audience seemed to absorb it a little more easily if you added in a dose of laughter. None of us found it that funny, but people tend to shut down and stop listening if all they hear is anger and accusation.

Our speakers' bureau training and meetings were fun, but they were also sad. Every time we got together there was always someone who was just a little sicker, who was just a little more tired, or who didn't look all that great. The worst part was the not knowing. Not knowing what was going on inside your body, not knowing if you were going to be the next one who didn't look so great. I kept looking around the room and wondering which one of these friends would be the next. The next to die.

In this scenario of people dying, we would share real-life problems and dilemmas, much of which was never shared with a larger audience. I remember people saying that they were just charging up their VISA bills because they didn't expect to live to have to pay the balance off. It's not like most of them were out there going on frivolous shopping sprees. Many were having to decide between paying their light bill or being able to feed the cat. The cat would win out 100 percent of the time.

Things like that were so sad, and everything in me wanted to fix things, to find solutions. But instead, I tried to listen and be compassionate, while occasionally delivering cat food.

A few on the speakers' bureau were couples where both people were infected, and both were speakers. It was heartbreaking when one person in a relationship began to have serious health issues and began to go downhill. I was glad that Scott was not infected, but, to be honest, in that group, it also gave me something to feel guilty about.

We did laugh a lot, and, like I said, not always about suitable things. One example about death that many of us used when we were speaking was that "Everyone is going to die; you never know when it's going to be your turn. I mean you could go outside today and get hit by a bus. You never know. "

Once in our monthly meeting, someone shared that a member of the Portland AIDS Speakers' Bureau had been hit by a bus. Inappropriately, we all burst out laughing. I mean, we knew that it wasn't funny someone had died, but the fact that we had been using that example forever ... let me just say that we stopped using the bus illustration.

People on the speakers' bureau were endearing. As they got sicker and literally were naming the few T cells they had left, people would ask more and more about me. How was I doing? These friends were generous, often offering what little they had to help another speaker. People were affectionate. Everyone hugged. Hugging and touching was a crucial part of our community. In a world where many were being rejected, touching was a necessity.

The speakers' bureau became an oasis for me. A safe place. A place to be honest and real. The people there changed my life, broke my narrow views, and expanded my horizons.

This began almost ten years of speaking about AIDS.

DEBBIE

There is nothing I would not do for those
who are really my friends.
I have no notion of loving people by halves;
it is not my nature.

Jane Austen, Northanger Abbey

f this story ever became a movie, one of the supporting actors would be my friend Debbie. I met Debbie when I was a sixth grader. She began to date my cousin, Pat, during her freshman year of high school. Pat was the same age as my brothers and sister and grew up in Bellevue, outside of Seattle.

In his college years, Pat and his friends came to our house in Wenatchee one spring for the Apple Blossom Festival. The festival, always a big party in town, boasted a parade and a lot of local festivities. Pat and Debbie showed up and pitched a few tents in our backyard for their friends. I was in junior high and lived alone with my parents, so Apple Blossom was exciting for me, especially having older kids at our house.

Back then, I only knew Debbie as a friend of my older siblings and my cousin, an almost grown-up who seemed way older than me but who still always took notice that I was there.

In August 1994, I heard from Dad that Pat and Debbie, now married with three kids, had moved to Spokane. This was great news because, until then, our closest relatives were about three hours by car. I was curious about where in Spokane they were, so I called the phone operator and asked for their number and then asked for the address. Back in the day, sometimes you could get the operator to give you an address, and sometimes they wouldn't. That day she did, and I noticed their house was less than a mile from mine.

I got in my car and drove to their new house. I was just going to do a drive-by but when I did, Debbie was standing right in the middle of the front yard, taking a break from carrying boxes into the house. She immediately spotted me. I pulled over and nonchalantly tried to pull off gracious and welcoming friend vibes despite feeling like I was the nosey younger cousin trying to tag along with the cool kids at Apple Blossom.

Little did I know this was the beginning of what would be one of the most important relationships in my entire life.

Debbie is a smart, positive, tiny person with a huge heart. I knew she was a loyal person because of the relationship I'd witnessed for years between her and Pat. I knew she was interested in healthcare because she had spent years working as a dietician in various healthcare settings. But what I learned while chatting with her that day on her front lawn was that Debbie also had a huge faith life that I knew nothing about. Neither of our families was particularly religious, and I didn't know any family member, other than Scott and me, who went to church.

During that initial conversation, Debbie told me she had signed up for a Bible study that met once a week in the community. I was already signed up, so I told her, "Let's go together." Debbie also joined my gym where I'd been doing a weightlifting program my sister had set up for me.

That fall, with the kids back in classes, Debbie and I fell

into a routine of dropping our kids off at school, then going to the gym, except on Tuesdays when we'd head to Bible study. From the beginning of Debbie moving to Spokane, we pretty much spent every day together.

If my public life with HIV was going to be a hike, then Debbie was going to be my hiking partner. Looking back, I'm incredibly thankful that I was given a best friend to help me navigate this now very public journey I was on.

SUPPORT GROUP

God sets the lonely in families.

Psalm 68:6

I'm not quite sure how our Christian AIDS support group came to be. I asked Debbie one day, "Why did we feel the need to have a Christian support group?" I added, somewhat facetiously, "To save souls?"

She immediately responded, "Always. In many different ways. People had no one who cared." Debbie was reminding me that apart from saving souls eternally, we were perhaps saving people from loneliness, providing a substitute family of sorts, a community that cared. What Debbie said was true, some people had no one who cared.

One of the speakers' bureau members, George, would say, "I've watched an enormous amount of people die in various ways. I've had several friends commit suicide over HIV and AIDS. That's a heartbreak. I've seen friends die in nursing homes and hospitals where the family doesn't even come to visit them. I've had friends who can't even go anywhere to die; they either lose their partners or their family."

After I'd been on the speakers' bureau for a few months I decided to put out an invitation to fellow speakers, telling them we were starting a support group with a spiritual bent. Immediately one of the group, Barry, asked in a very cynical voice, "Is this a *Christian* thing?"

I didn't want to lie or be misleading: "Well, yes, I guess we're all Christians who are setting up the group."

A few days after the invite, Barry called me, with a very angry voice. Barry wasn't talking to me on the phone; he was yelling at me. He didn't hold back in saying I was a terrible person and that I was not helping but actually adding to the problem of HIV and the church. Barry felt that by having a "Christian" support group, we were excluding all other kinds of faith groups, and he was worried his friends would, once again, feel rejected and hurt.

I'd known that the church and religion remained sensitive topics for a lot of people who were living with AIDS. People who had been shunned and excluded, even chastised by the church. Many were told that their illness was God's judgment on their lives and choices. I, of course, had no intention of making that prejudice and stigma worse. The other leaders of this group and I weren't intending to open those wounds and create pain for people. Barry felt like we were doing just that.

We tossed around the idea of calling it a "faith" group, a more general and more inclusive name, but we didn't want to misrepresent the fact that all of us who were leading the group were Christians, having a traditional Christian faith. We didn't want people to feel lied to or manipulated.

On the other hand, we truly weren't meaning to exclude any other faith or belief system. Looking back, it may have been a mistake to label it anything other than a group for "support," and it did take several sensitive conversations before we were being viewed as an accepting, open group that cared.

In the end, I appreciated the angry call from Barry, although it made me feel a bit unliked and unwelcomed by our speakers' bureau. It was good to check my intentions and think about the pain others experienced in the name of God.

But I did wonder where all of Barry's irritation was coming from. I mean, I understood his concern, but the amount of outrage seemed over the top. I remember thinking, "Why is this straight guy so mad?" Barry was a hemophiliac, so it didn't seem like he was talking from his own experience.

Well, like most things that at first don't make sense, Barry's anger toward religion *was*, it turns out, from his own experience. As I got to know Barry better, I heard his story. Barry grew up in St. Louis, in a Catholic family. He graduated from St. Louis University and went on to become a Jesuit priest and teacher. After joining the order, his superiors found out he had HIV, and he was released from his position. He petitioned to proceed to ordination but was denied. Barry left the priesthood, later getting married. I love the quote from Barry when he was interviewed in *POZ Magazine*. "People ask me if I left God when I left the order," Barry said. "But I believe that God is bigger than the Jesuits."

I couldn't have agreed with him more.

As I got to know Barry better, I noticed that he poured most of his energy into three things: raising his daughter, being an artist, and advocating for a financial settlement for HIV-positive hemophiliacs. Barry was passionate and often communicated with seriousness and intensity. I found that his passion could sometimes be misunderstood as anger.

Our support group met off and on for a couple of years. Usually, we'd meet at one of our houses or at Scott's office. The group time was more about sharing and eating than any kind of Bible study. We usually ended by asking what everyone wanted us to pray for, and then someone would pray, often Scott. It was almost always the same people who came: Debbie, my friend Carolyn, and occasionally her husband, Ed, Scott, and myself. We were joined by a few people from our speakers' bureau: Joyce, Camie, Craig, and, once in a while, George and Barry.

George, an HIV-positive Lutheran minister who became a mentor and friend to me, only came to our support group a couple of times. The last time he showed up I drove him home to his place in Browne's Addition and as he was getting out of my car he paused and looked at me. He was standing there quietly like he was collecting his thoughts and then he said, "What you're doing matters." He smiled at me and went into his house.

It was a huge endorsement of our measly efforts, trying to love and take care of people, trying to help find a bigger purpose, a bigger family, a family when there wasn't family, a family that included God.

These were the people who would end up being my core friends with HIV. Others came and went at the speakers' bureau, and I loved getting to know them and hearing their stories, but this AIDS Support Group crew grew to be much more to me than mere acquaintances or colleagues. We became dear friends and made a point to have each other's backs. To provide food and transportation when one of us was stuck. To listen and to laugh ... deeply. To sit at someone's bedside, again and again. To advocate at the hospital for water, food, blankets, painkillers, comfort, attention, whatever was needed—making sure no one was ignored or treated poorly.

These were my people, my friends with AIDS who loved me and knew me.

THE BLIND SKIER

If I see anything vital around me,
it is precisely that spirit of adventure,
which seems indestructible and is akin to curiosity.

Marie Curie

first met Carolyn through Kristine, and she became Ryan's special person. I remember picking Ryan up from her house; he was about three years old, and Carolyn had set up a TV tray where he ate lunch looking out her living room window at the road construction happening outside. Ryan was mesmerized, engrossed in all the activity and people in yellow and orange hard hats working just steps away.

Carolyn and her husband, Ed, were excited to be part of the team who helped and attended our support group. Carolyn, a professional counselor with a soft voice and an equally caring heart, put people at ease. Her brother lived in Seattle and had been battling AIDS for some time. That relationship and experience gave her a desire to support the HIV community in Spokane.

Carolyn's family formed a strong bond with Craig, one of my speakers' bureau friends who regularly came to our support group. Craig was a young, good-looking guy with a ginger complexion, strawberry hair, and a sweet smile to match. Craig and I instantly got along, but then it seemed like Craig connected with pretty much everyone.

Craig was very committed to our support group; I'm pretty sure he never missed a meeting and showed up at almost every event we planned. He hung out often with Carolyn and Ed and loved being with their family, even tagging along to church on Sundays and eventually becoming like a favorite relative, occasionally joining them on vacations.

Craig had stories. At times we'd all have to wonder how many of them were real, partially real, or imagined. One thing was certain, they were entertaining. Craig once told me that he was bisexual, saying he had been married to a woman from a rich family in Texas. He boasted about his twin boys born out of that relationship. He explained that pressure from her family forced him to give up custody after he came out. There were no photos of the boys and the story changed intermittently to fit whatever circumstances Craig found himself in. I just listened most of the time and nodded a lot instead of saying much.

The truth was, I didn't put a lot of thought or judgment into any of these tales; there were so many stories; many very sad, many grandiose, many contradictory. All I knew for sure was that Craig didn't have any family nearby, and his friends were very important to him.

Craig was in good physical condition for the most part except for one major thing: he was going blind from cytomegalovirus, an opportunistic infection that damages the eyes of those who are immunocompromised. The crazy thing was that he got a housing allotment from the State of Washington for being blind while still being issued a Washington State driver's license. The contradiction summed up Craig in general—he was a person with a whole lot of things that just didn't quite go together. Nevertheless, I loved hanging out with him and learned it was best to just not ask questions.

I used to tease Craig that he was a great shopping companion. He couldn't give me a bad time about anything I was buying because he couldn't see—and we always got the best parking spots, even during the Christmas rush, with his handicap parking pass. Craig was often available to go on a drive, so I would pick him up while I was running errands. He loved getting out of the house while his roommates were at work, and I enjoyed having another adult to talk to.

One of the funniest things that Craig asked me to do was to teach him how to cross-country ski. By then he was almost completely blind. He was so sincere about the request, so I put my mind to how we could pull this off without hurting him or anyone else in the process.

Carolyn and Ed lived on a farm a ways out of town, and that winter Spokane had a fair amount of snow. I asked Carolyn if we could come out and try to ski down some of her rolling hills. Luckily, Craig was the same shoe size as Scott, so we had the right equipment to make this happen.

I knew that if Craig were to ski safely, we'd have to remove all barriers and dangers. I went out in advance to try to tap down some of the snow and figure out a place where we wouldn't be running into barbed wire fences and things like that. Really, what it came down to was that Craig wanted to go straight downhill as fast as he could and get the feeling of just being free. Fortunately, he was a strong young man who could absorb the eventual and predictable crash that came at the end of each run.

Off he went, over and over falling headlong, sideways, and every way imaginable for hours until we were both freezing, and I had run out of energy from continually collecting all of his gear. Craig crashed all day, followed by tons and tons of laughter and joy. I'll never forget that magical day.

CAMIE
AND WORLD AIDS DAY

Let your life lightly dance on the edges of time
like dew on the tip of a leaf.

Rabindranath Tagore

The Spokane AIDS Network sometimes put on informational meetings focused on women who were infected and affected by AIDS. In the early days, several women attended these educational sessions, but only a few of us were HIV-positive, including Joyce, Camie, and myself.

Both Joyce and Camie were single moms. Joyce had kids the same age as mine, even though she was five years younger than me. Camie, on the other hand, was about the same age as Joyce but had a much younger child, a two-year-old.

At first, Camie seemed to be a wholesome schoolgirl type with quiet charm and a youthful demeanor—that was, until she opened her mouth and revealed a more complex woman with a seriously sassy spirit. When I met her, I was instantly impressed with her intelligence and wit. But, as I was around her more, I decided that her most endearing characteristic was her tears. There wasn't a meeting or a speaking engagement where she wouldn't cry. Unlike me, she could cry and talk at the same time. She could laugh and cry at the same time. She could tell a joke and cry at the same time. She wore her heart on her sleeve, and it was impossible not to be drawn to her.

I enjoyed Camie immensely. She was a perfect ally in what became a trio, our HIV girls club. She and Joyce both welcomed me as the third musketeer.

Camie was a loving and dedicated mom; her two-year-old was her life. She was living in a small apartment she could barely afford and wasn't receiving public assistance at the time, so every spare dime she earned on the speakers' bureau went to her son, to make his life the best it could be. Camie seemed very aware that her time with him was ticking away. Watching them broke my heart.

I have to say, as much as I knew I could die soon, I never felt the urgency I saw in Camie. I didn't see that urgency in Joyce either. I think Joyce and I still held out hope for a future, whereas Camie seemed very in touch with her limited timeline.

Camie was once quoted in a newspaper article after speaking to some junior high parents. I was so proud to know her when I read it. She was a very brave woman, a courageous mother who shared what she wanted her young son to know and say about her.

> "I want him to be honest," she said. "I want him to say, 'My mother died of AIDS, but she was courageous and strong.'"
>
> "I don't want him to pay for what happened to me ... I may die from this disease," she said. "But this disease will not defeat me."
>
> *Spokesman Review*, February 18, 1995

Every year the speakers' bureau helped shape and put together a community program on World AIDS Day, December 1. Usually, the event included some of our speakers sharing reflections and a remembrance of people who'd been lost, with friends and family solemnly naming loved ones who had died of AIDS and everyone lighting candles in a vigil.

1994 was my first World AIDS Day since becoming a speaker. I'd been to events in the past, but I'd been anonymous and didn't know anyone. This year it took on new significance in two ways: I was now part of the community, and I knew some of the people who had died.

That year the event and vigil were scheduled to be at Manito Park, outside. I'm not sure who had thought this was a good location; Spokane is known for its very cold weather, and early December is often frigid. The idea to gather up all the sick people with compromised immune systems and stick them outside on a dark winter evening, in hindsight, was not smart. But it was World AIDS Day, our only day. Some diseases get whole months of recognition, but HIV and AIDS only have one day, December 1.

Manito Park is quite expansive with a large pond in the center. I mention this because on that cold night, the pond turned into a real problem for Camie. Other than the night being freezing cold, causing us all to huddle close to control our shivering, the event had been going well until the sound of a splash sent every parent within earshot into overdrive. Camie's two-year-old had fallen into the partially frozen pond. Acting at lightning speed, several of us fetched him out of the water, took him to a warm car, and dried him off. We found some dry clothes and thought that was the end of it.

A few days later Camie got very sick, apparently from the pond water at Manito. She had been exposed to cryptosporidium, a bacteria that wreaks havoc on the intestinal tract of anyone with a compromised immune system. From that day on, Camie found it very hard to keep food down. We didn't know it at the time, but it would be the beginning of her undoing.

Her health would not recover.

A HAMBURGER

A strong woman
knows she has strength for the journey,
but a woman of strength knows
that it is in the journey where she will become strong.

Unknown

few weeks after fishing a small child out of a freezing pond, Joyce and Camie told me they were going to go to Washington, D.C., to one of the first conventions for women with AIDS. Having signed up in advance, they had received scholarships and everything was set up for them. I wanted to go too, not wanting to be the one in our trio who was left out, especially since it was specifically for women! But, by the time I heard about the conference, it was just a couple of weeks away and I wasn't sure how to pull off attending. Then Scott's dad, my wonderful father-in-law, offered to pay my way, even at the very high, last minute, prices. So, I signed up, booked a hotel room, and prepared to go to D.C.

The Second Conference on HIV Infection in Women was held in Washington, D.C., from February 22 through 24, 1995. This was Wednesday through Friday, but we stayed in the District until Sunday afternoon. Besides the actual sessions at the conference, we were also scheduled to talk to our legislators on Capitol Hill.

At the beginning of the AIDS epidemic, women were excluded from advocacy, treatment, and research. Women were blocked from being subjects in clinical trials even into the early 1990s, especially if they were of childbearing age or could possibly be pregnant. This meant that women, and children, were being prescribed drugs for HIV infection that had never been tested, or had undergone very limited testing, on women (almost none on kids). The National Institutes of Health rejected grants that were targeted at understanding HIV in low-income women of ethnic minorities, and in 1987 allowed only 13.5 percent of their budget to be allocated to women's health issues in general. This discrimination was despite the fact that worldwide, by 1988, the number of women infected with HIV in other areas of the world was very high; in sub-Saharan Africa, HIV infection in women was higher than in men. At that time in the US, the idea that women were being infected with HIV seemed like an afterthought.

Finally, in 1992, the Centers for Disease Control expanded the definition of HIV to include symptoms experienced by people of color and women who were in HIV trials and treatment. After the definition was changed, immediately the number of women with AIDS in the US increased by 50 percent. Women were finally being counted and were subsequently eligible for Medicare and Social Security benefits that had previously been denied. By 1993, AIDS had become the leading cause of death for African-American women aged twenty-two to forty-four.

Women and their kids who had been infected, some of whom were dying of AIDS, were asking for equal treatment, equal access, and the recognition that women and families had unique symptoms and needs within the AIDS community. We were going to D.C. to lobby on behalf of these families, and ourselves.

Our first goal was to learn as much as we could about HIV and women, including new and promising treatments. Our second goal was personal. Ever since Camie fetched her child out of the pond on World AIDS Day, she'd been dealing with a vicious intestinal infection that was making it difficult to keep food down, and she was losing weight. Her doctor told her that if things didn't change, she would soon be put on TPN, artificial food given through a tube. Camie was struggling to afford these treatments because, even though she was very ill, she had been denied Social Security Disability and Medicare coverage several times.

The three of us were going to march straight up Capitol Hill to ask all of our Washington State elected congressional representatives to help Camie get coverage. It seemed like an achievable goal, and we were armed with our personal stories and photos of all seven of our beautiful children.

The information being presented at the conference was a bit overwhelming; I'd never been to a scientific gathering on this scale before. One thing that was new to me was the presence of ACT UP, the AIDS Coalition to Unleash Power. ACT UP, started in 1987 by Larry Kramer, strove to improve the lives and treatment of people with AIDS through direct action, medical research, treatment, and advocacy by working to change legislation and public policies. They often used civil disobedience to get their message across. In Washington, D.C., that year a large contingent of ACT UP protesters were doing just that: acting up.

To be honest, I had mixed feelings about the protesters at the time because they were disrupting the conference, the one my father-in-law had paid for that I wanted to get a lot out of. But the more I learned, the more I understood clearly that I probably wouldn't have even been sitting in such a conference without their efforts on behalf of people living with HIV, especially women.

The next day we went to Capitol Hill to meet with George Nethercutt, our representative from Spokane. We showed him our photos and told him our stories. When I told George my cousin Debbie's sister lived right next door to him, he looked uncomfortable, like AIDS had come just a little too close to home.

The highlight of the day was when one of Nethercutt's aides told us he was determined to get Camie on Medicare. Lo and behold, he kept his promise. Within a few weeks, she was accepted.

That night, the last night the three of us were together, we were exhausted from traversing a strange city, navigating the metro, getting lost in the endless hallways of government buildings, not to mention the mental and emotional weight of sharing our stories again and again. The only thing I was looking forward to was one more night of uninterrupted sleep in a hotel room. Camie had other ideas.

"Are we going out?" Joyce and I looked at her—surely she was joking? Sensing our bewilderment, she added, "To get some drinks?"

Camie had a youthful spirit that sometimes made Joyce and me feel like old ladies. After we'd been lobbying the whole day and going to conference seminars, going for drinks was, for Joyce and me, literally the last thing on our minds.

We both took deep breaths and with less than a little enthusiasm replied, "Sure."

Camie, one way or another, always reminded us that we were still young, that it was just our bodies that were betraying us. We went back to the hotel, got ourselves "bar ready," and went out on the town.

Suddenly, we felt young again.

Finding a lively Irish pub, we ate, we drank, and we pretended we were normal gals. We didn't talk about AIDS. We just wanted a night off from it all.

At one point, Camie, who'd hardly been able to hold down food for weeks, ordered a giant hamburger, fries, and a beer. Joyce and I looked at each other with an equal amount of surprise and concern.

Then Camie said, "This is probably the last full meal I'll ever eat."

She was right. That was one of the last meals I ever saw her eat. But the look of enjoyment on her face convinced me that she knew exactly what she was doing.

NEW HOPE

. Just living is not enough ...
one must have sunshine, freedom, and a little flower.

Hans Christian Andersen

One day, in the fall of 1995, I burst into Dr. C's office and, with a smile, announced, "Hey, I've outlived your prediction!"

"What in the world are you talking about?" he asked with a furrowed brow.

I reminded him that at our first appointment, he had predicted that I had three to five years to live. "This is my five-year anniversary!"

He chuckled and said, "What kind of crazy doctor would say that?" Then added, "I really knew nothing at that time about life expectancy with HIV. Maybe none of us did. I would give you way more than that now. Many, many more years."

It was a great day to let that "three to five" go.

Years later, I asked Debbie if, in the mid-1990s, I'd still thought I was going to die.

"I remember during that time you and Scott were looking into buying a house at the end of the Moran Prairie playground" (our kids' school). "I remember," she said, "you saying that when you got so sick that you would need to be in a wheelchair, you could sit on the back patio and watch your kids play at recess."

It came back to me, that memory, but had totally forgotten. In the moment of her reminding me, it felt like she was talking about someone else's life at some other time. But it was my life, my feelings, and my fears. The outcome and life expectancy for people with HIV were about to change drastically in the next few years, but when I was living it, those days still seemed far away and not a guarantee for everyone who was HIV-positive.

Two things significantly changed my medical treatment and prognosis in the mid-1990s. First of all, a new class of medications for HIV, called protease inhibitors, came out of drug trials for use in the general HIV population. These drugs could be combined with antiretrovirals to fight the infection from different phases of the life cycle of HIV. Suddenly T cells were going up and viral load, or the amount of virus in a person's body, was going down. People were becoming healthier. These new drugs were not without their own side effects, but still, they were a light at the end of the tunnel, new hope that we might live more days in what had been a dismal future forecast.

People began to ask me, "Are you in remission?"

I would explain that remission, like what happens to people being treated for cancer, is not a thing with HIV. With HIV, every day my body is making millions of copies of HIV, and every day my body is destroying millions of copies of HIV. HIV-positive people continue to stay healthy by keeping this in balance; that's what the drugs are for. The minute the body gets worn down and cannot keep up with destroying the virus, HIV builds up in the body and a person's immune system starts to suffer.

The goal is to manage HIV, to keep the virus at levels that are "undetectable." This doesn't mean the virus is gone; it means it is so low that the test cannot detect it. If a person stops HIV medications, eventually the test will be able to detect HIV because it will, again, over time build up in the body.

Undetectable HIV is the goal. That is a simplified version of what the medications do.

The second thing that happened about the same time that the new medicines came on the scene was that I changed doctors. I had loved going to Dr. C, but he was a pulmonologist and we both agreed that the treatment protocol was getting more complicated and sophisticated so it would be better if I saw an infectious disease specialist who focused primarily on HIV. At the time, there were two such physicians in Spokane. I chose one who would be my doctor for the next six years.

I was surprised to learn that my new physician had informed the Washington State Department of Health that I had an official AIDS diagnosis from a chronic yeast infection I had experienced a couple of years earlier. I had no idea that esophageal candidiasis, yeast in your throat, was on the list of AIDS-defining conditions. This didn't really change anything for me personally, but our state received HIV treatment and care funding based on the number of people whose HIV infection had progressed to AIDS. If an AIDS diagnosis meant more money for our community, I was all for it!

In some ways, this new AIDS diagnosis felt like defeat, but, in other ways, it felt a bit liberating. I had to admit that, even with all my effort, the disease had progressed. Maybe it was better to let it go a bit. Either I was going to live or die, and, apparently, I was not going to be the one to choose which scenario would win out. I began to understand why some people take their own life at the time they choose. It's about many things, I suppose, but I think one of those is getting to be the one to choose. To have some control when everything else seems out of control.

I decided to be positive while trying to not be so focused on control. I began to think more and more about purposeful living and enjoying life. Yet friends around me continued to die.

This was survival, and almost everyone I knew with HIV and AIDS was trying to live in this paradox.

CASSEROLES ...
CHURCH LADIES

Aunt Fidelia
Brought the rolls
With her
Green bean casserole
The widow Smith
Down the street
Dropped by a bowl
Of butter beans
Plastic cups
And silverware
Lime green
Tupperware everywhere
Pass the chicken
Pass the pie
We sure eat good
When someone dies

Kate Campbell

E ven with the new protocol of meds with the protease inhibitors, and help from a naturopath, I was still having bouts of sickness, achiness, and difficulty getting going many days. Adding public speaking a few days a week left me exhausted. After sharing this with a Bible study that I'd been a part of for the last few years, the small group of women offered their help by way of making and delivering dinner for our family a night or two a week. And help it was, especially on days when I was speaking at a school out of town and half of my day was spent driving to and from the speaking engagement.

I loved this Bible study, and I like to think of the women in it as the younger, cooler version of the typical "church lady," helping me feed my family so I could continue to drive around Eastern Washington teaching teens about HIV, STDs, and the importance of safe sex. I was absolutely grateful for the support.

Being the type of person who likes it when food doesn't touch on a dinner plate, I was never a huge fan of casseroles, and they weren't something I regularly made for my kids. But more than that, we were all just trying to have a semi-regular life, and then suddenly, someone would show up with food, the type of thing my kids knew we did for our own very sick friends from time to time.

I don't want to seem ungrateful. I did consider these meals helpful and truly appreciated that they took care of one thing that I wouldn't have to think about and plan for on days when I was exhausted. Unfortunately, what my kids were experiencing was a disconnect between our day-to-day life, which seemed semi-normal, and the reality that their mom was sick and could die. To them, church ladies bringing dinners to our house supported the "my mom is dying" storyline. There's even a casserole to back up their feelings— "Funeral Potatoes," made of hashbrowns and topped with cornflakes, popular at funeral luncheons across the Midwest.

And, just practically, casseroles weren't what they liked or usually ate. However, I wasn't going to complain. My friends were truly stepping up to help.

So, this is how it came to be that a couple of nights each week, a Ford Explorer or perhaps a Dodge Caravan would pull up to our house. A well-meaning friend would climb out, clad in stirrup pants or a tracksuit with a coordinating turtleneck. She'd weave her way up the front walk, around miscellaneous bikes and rollerblades, modes of transportation for visiting neighbor kids who hadn't yet gone to their own homes for dinner. She'd ring the doorbell, covered casserole dish in hand, notecard taped to the top with the correct heating instructions written out in perfect cursive.

One of those afternoons I was within earshot of Laura running to the door to intercept one of these deliveries.

The kind woman delivering food said very enthusiastically, "Hi Laura, I have dinner here for you!"

Laura, with no enthusiasm: "Is it a casserole?"

"Yes!" the kind woman replied, offering the dish out for Laura to take, oblivious to her disdain.

Blocking the doorway, Laura, my child blessed with the gift of brutal honesty, blurted, "I hate casseroles."

Then she abruptly turned and walked away, leaving the woman at the door, mouth agape, casserole still in hand.

I immediately intervened with the most cheerful, grateful, and apologetic dialogue I could muster. I was so embarrassed.

I tried not to be mad. This was hard to know how to reconcile and harder still to explain to the Bible study the next week. They were like, "Do you still want dinners? Is it helpful?"

There was a principle at work here. Something that we could see if we just took a step back from what was actually happening and tried to understand *why* it was happening, what was underneath.

Casseroles were the enemy, especially to this child whose

main defense and survival tactic had always been denial. The people who brought them were not her friends. To her, they were hastening my descent into the grave. She was an eleven-year-old. None of this was conscious on her part. Laura would've rather made herself a peanut butter and jelly sandwich for dinner than eat any delivered meal, no matter what it was.

I canceled the dinners.

I'm often asked for advice on how to help a sick friend. Thank God for the variety of food delivery services that exist now, where a family can decide on their own what to eat. But really, if your generosity doesn't land the way that you hoped, don't take it personally. For families dealing with sickness, there's often much more going on under the surface. I'm still a strong believer that it's better to try to do something than to do nothing at all, even if it goes sideways; the family will know you care—and *that* is worth more than you'll ever know.

COLORADO SPRINGS

I like your Christ, I do not like your Christians.
Your Christians are so unlike your Christ.

Gandhi

D uring that season, when my women's Bible study was bringing over food, Carolyn moved to Seattle and stayed on Capitol Hill to be near a skilled nursing home specifically for people with AIDS called Bailey Boushay House. The thirty-five-bed facility was built in 1992 because hospitals in the Seattle area didn't have enough space or skills to deal with the growing number of people dying of AIDS. Carolyn was there to care for her brother, Chuck, who was in his last days. Sadly, he died on St. Patrick's Day.

After she returned to Spokane, Carolyn and I decided to attend a Christian AIDS conference in Colorado Springs. I'm not sure how we heard about this gathering or what enticed us to go; maybe we wanted our own AIDS support group to have more resources. We have varied memories of that trip but one thing we both remember was a large contingent of folks from Exodus International with an underlying theme that they could "pray the gay away."

In the mid-1990s, Colorado, and particularly Colorado Springs, was a divided entity when it came to human rights issues regarding gay, lesbian, and bisexual discrimination. A biased and judgmental attitude had spilled over in some of the churches' view of people with HIV and AIDS in general.

In November of 1992, the state had approved by initiative an amendment to the Colorado state constitution, Amendment 2, that would prevent any city, town, or county in the state from taking any legislative, executive, or judicial action to recognize homosexuals or bisexuals as a protected class. Backers portrayed it as outlawing special rights for gays, lesbians, and bisexuals, which, in turn, provoked outrage nationwide and branded Colorado the "Hate State."

Voters set in motion a legal and constitutional fight when they approved it. After a highly public battle discussed regularly on conservative TV shows by the likes of Pat Robertson and his Christian Coalition, in 1996 the US Supreme Court deemed Amendment 2 unconstitutional. By the time Carolyn and I attended the Christian AIDS conference, the stage had been set for the evangelical Christians in Colorado Springs, the home of James Dobson's Focus on the Family, to view the LGBTQ community as enemies of the church and a threat to conservative views of gender and sexual relationships.

At the conference, about 150 people sat in rows listening to speakers who discussed the evils of homosexuality and the judgment of God in the form of AIDS, and how we needed to love the sinner and hate the sin. There was no angry passion or dramatic ranting. It all was discussed calmly with sugary smooth talk. It occurred to me that this is the sly way discrimination is spread, with a calm smile and a sincere prayer.

From the moment we understood that the conference was cloaked in homophobia and judgment, rather than simply caring for people with AIDS, we were frustrated and concerned. For me, it was a hard weekend and a turning point. I couldn't imagine my brother being different than he was, and I didn't buy in to the idea that somehow a gay person could change their sexuality or identity. No way was I going to pray for him to change who he was born to be.

Looking back to that weekend in Colorado, this wasn't the beginning of my disagreement with many Christians and with the evangelical church around issues of sexual orientation and gender identity, but it was the beginning of being vocal about that disagreement. As I began to vocalize those thoughts, I found that in the years following, I received fewer and fewer invitations to speak and share my story in churches. I had become controversial, a bit of a liability.

I was no longer safe to the very people who had been my faith community.

KARA

The people who influence us most are
not those who buttonhole us and talk to us,
but those who live their lives like the stars in the
heavens and the lilies in the field,
perfectly, simply and unaffectedly.
Those are the lives that mold us.

Oswald Chambers

During spring break in 1995, we took a family trip to Disneyland. Ryan was just tall enough, with a pair of thick-soled shoes and standing as straight as he could, to go on the brand-new Indiana Jones ride. The ride had opened a couple of weeks earlier, and the lines were incredibly long. But, it was his birthday, and that ride was the one thing he wanted to do most of all. I volunteered to stand in line with him for two and a half hours, snaking through the maze that Disney created to entertain the masses lined up. This was back in the theme park dark ages, before the "fast-pass" was invented. Most of the enjoyment for me was just watching Ryan have one of his seven-year-old dreams fulfilled.

That trip provided a break from our day-to-day, and being in the California sun felt glorious. Looking back, glancing at photos from that trip, including ones of me crashing and snoozing poolside, I do remember that even vacations took all of my strength.

We came home to the news that Joyce's daughter, Kara, was continuing to become weaker and having trouble fighting infections that were constantly attacking her system.

That winter, Kara had been hospitalized a couple of times. Kara celebrated her seventh birthday on April 1 that year and we all attended, teasing her about being an April Fool's baby. The contrast between Ryan's seventh birthday a week earlier, watching him run around Disneyland, and Kara's celebration smack dab in the middle of hospitalizations and her small body doing its best to hang on, was not lost on any of us. It reminded me of how truly unfair things can be and how little we have to say about living and dying, even when it's a child.

That would be her last birthday. On April Fool's Day the next year, the same group would meet to have cake and candles; we would even sing the birthday song— but there would not be an eight-year-old to blow out the candles.

In June of 1995, the local newspaper did a story about Kara's first grade school year. They summarized what a brutal year it had been on Kara's health, highlighting how, even through it all, she still held on to her warm and loving spirit:

> She missed 40 days of school. She was hospitalized three times that winter, first for infected sinuses, then twice for herpes zoster, the virus that causes chickenpox. In April, Joyce took her to Seattle Children's Hospital and Medical Center. The doctors there changed Kara's medicines.
>
> She moves more slowly and looks smaller and paler than her Willard Elementary classmates. Her doctor said she hasn't gained weight in two years. She takes seven

different medications that boost her immune system and keep chronic infections at bay. But AIDS dismantled her body's natural defense during the past eighteen months and now she stands vulnerable to germs most people shake off without a cough ... "She is still stubborn, funny, and sparkling. She gives me joy and memories I'll always have, that sense of honor and admiration that someone so young can be so strong and tenacious," said Mrs. Hammond, who will teach Kara again next fall.

"At one point this winter when she wasn't doing well, she said to me, 'Mrs. Hammond, the end is really close,'" said her teacher. "All I could do was give her a hug. I couldn't say, 'Oh, it's not.' That wouldn't be an honest answer."

Spokesman Review, June 19, 1995

In July, Kara suffered from fevers and headaches that wouldn't go away. On July 21, Joyce brought her to Deaconess Medical Center. On July 25, they discovered a lesion in her brain, but no one knew quite what it was although further testing showed it was destroying Kara's normal brain tissue. Joyce and the boys moved into Kara's hospital room in early August.

The kids and I made regular visits to the hospital that August. Joyce welcomed the distraction and help in not only entertaining Kara, but also having friends for her boys to hang out with.

Kara had a particular favorite toy, a magic wand, which

she almost always had on hand to turn you into various objects or animals or to say what she was wishing for. One thing she hated was her pink medicine and had a strong clenched jaw when she refused to take it. The pink medicine was something we spent a great deal of time brainstorming about, coming up with bribes good enough to get her to open her mouth and slurp it down.

Some days after visiting, we'd bring the boys, Dale and Chris, home with us overnight, and once we took them to Priest Lake for a few days. Dale was definitely worried about Kara and talked a little about his feelings, but Chris never said a word about his sister and would usually leave the room if the subject of Kara's health or the hospital came up.

It was hard not to internalize what was happening to this little girl. I was so aware that what the Claypools were going through could have easily been our story. Ryan's due date was Kara's actual birthday, April 1. He was born a week early. They were both born to HIV-positive mothers. There was no intervention at the time. They both had a 25-30 percent chance of being born HIV-positive. He was lucky. She was not.

It's as simple as that.

I was at home when I got the call: "Come quickly, Kara doesn't have much more time." It was early in the morning on August 30, 1995, a few days before Kara was slated to start second grade.

I remember getting dressed. I purposely wore a T-shirt that had a cat face on the front of it with a Bible verse. I don't remember what the verse was. I picked that shirt because it was Joyce's favorite, and, as far as I was concerned, this day was going to be her day. Kara was going to die; Joyce was the one who would need me—she would need everyone.

When I arrived at Deaconess Hospital, several family

members and friends had settled in Kara's room. Chris played video games down the hall, and Dale greeted people as they came in the door. Joyce, lying on Kara's bed with her unresponsive body in her arms, talked sweetly to her and sang songs. I crossed the room and gave both of them a kiss. It was hard to take in what was actually happening, but Joyce seemed at complete peace.

Kara died in the late morning. Afterward, their minister, Pastor Smith, had everyone join hands in a circle and different people offered up prayers. Then Joyce began to sing hymns and those who knew the words joined in. I remember this like it was yesterday because somehow a photo of the whole scene ended up in the newspaper, solidifying it in my mind.

As the morning wore on, people began to leave. They said their condolences to Joyce and sometimes to the boys and then departed. I reminded myself that I was there for Joyce and would see this day through to the end, doing whatever she needed. As the coolness of that August morning turned to a bright sunny afternoon, we were still waiting for the funeral home to come and move Kara's body.

Joyce looked exhausted, needing a change of scenery from this room she had lived in for months and her lifeless seven-year-old's body. She looked over with soulful eyes. "Do you want to go to the roof?"

We made our way to the fresh air, her favorite smoking place since the hospital had become her home. Looking out over Spokane, her eyes brightened and she smiled. "Oh, wow, you wore my favorite shirt."

"Of course," I answered, pleased she had noticed. "I can't believe she's gone, Joyce." I blinked back tears.

"But she is with her dad and Jesus, and isn't in pain," Joyce reminded me, always focusing on her Jesus. "She is finally healed."

I replied with something to the effect that one great thing about when we die is that this bitch of a virus finally gets what's coming to it. This made her smile even more.

Kara finally was transferred to the mortuary where she would be cremated. I then did my best to talk Joyce into going home and getting some rest. The boys had been taken earlier by relatives. She finally quit resisting and began to say her goodbyes. It had to be the hardest thing to leave that room, her world, not for just the last few weeks but for the last several years. The nurses were visually upset and did not hold back tears in their goodbyes when Joyce finally walked down the hall and out the door.

Another friend and I stayed behind to pack up Kara's things. Cleaning out her room was quite a task because the whole family had been living there. Joyce had used a fold-out bed, and the boys had slept on mattresses in the corner of the room. There was a lot of accumulated stuff.

Packing that room added to the sadness of the day. It felt so final. I packed up Kara's life into boxes and wondered where those would end up. I was heartbroken. I loved this little girl, and I think all of us believed she would just keep going despite the odds. All that remained was a few boxes of "stuff." The stuff was meaningless without the seven-year-old it belonged to.

Then I found her magic wand; it was devastating to see. That magic wand belonged with Kara, like an extension of her arm.

Her life had been magical and way too short.

The next day I opened the *Spokesman Review* to the front-page headline, "Spokane Loses Littlest Hero."

Seven-year-old Kara Claypool died wrapped
in her mother's arms Wednesday in her bed

at Spokane's Deaconess Medical Center. Before slipping into a coma, she said, "I love you, Mom."

Joyce Claypool, smiling like the mother of a newborn, thanked God for answering prayers that her youngest child would have an easy death.

"My daughter is in heaven, safe and sound," she said.

Spokesman Review, August 31, 1995

Immediately the chain link fence at Willard Elementary School, Kara's school, began filling with flowers, ribbons, and handwritten messages. It became a memorial of sorts, where people from the greater community could express their love and admiration for this young life taken too soon. Joyce watched the memorial grow, driving by often and commenting on how many people loved her daughter.

A couple of days later, the school year started. Teresa was in sixth grade, Laura in fourth, and Ryan in second. Looking at the traditional "first day of school" picture I snapped that year on our front porch, I recall being a mess of mixed emotions. On one hand, I wanted my kids' lives to go on normally. But we had just witnessed a devastating loss, all of us helping to take care of this other family who had lost a child. On that day, that family, too, had a sixth grader and a fourth grader doing their best to get themselves to the first day of school. But instead of their second grader, Kara, sitting with her classmates, there would be an empty desk.

CIGARETTES
IN THE GARAGE

Come back. Even as a shadow, even as a dream.

Euripides

We all knew Kara was dying and that she probably wouldn't live to get out of grade school. We can believe we're prepared for something; we can plan and we can think about it and we can decide how we think we're going to respond. But nothing really prepares anyone to watch a child die. Especially if it's your own child.

The first few days after Kara's death, Joyce was so positive. She talked about Jesus a lot. She talked about Kara being with her dad in heaven. She gave interviews to the press. She sang songs and tried to find all of the blessings in having been Kara's mom for seven years.

And then she plunged headlong into a deep, sad depression.

Joyce stopped functioning. I stopped by her house, and her oldest son, Dale, was the one keeping things going. He kept the family fed by going to the store and trying to get his brother to go to school. It was clear Dale and Chris hadn't gone to school much, and Joyce was barely getting dressed. One day I got a call from a mutual friend who asked if I would take all three of them to our home for a little while and make sure the kids got to school. So that day, I went to Joyce's house, packed her up, along with Chris and Dale, and moved them temporarily to our house.

When the Claypool family moved in, my plan was to get the boys to school, allowing Joyce the space to rest and wrap her head around life without Kara, to grieve and begin to process.

The weather turned rainy, and Joyce spent much of her time in our garage, with the door raised, smoking cigarettes. It was pretty much the only covered "smoking porch" I could provide, and Joyce loved her cigarettes, about one an hour.

I will admit, I was kind of embarrassed that Joyce was sitting in my garage with the garage door open smoking all the time. I don't know why this image bothered me. I guess, looking back, I tried to convey a certain type of lifestyle to my neighbors, and chain-smoking in the garage didn't fit that. It seems pretty stupid and petty thinking back on it now.

At the end of their second week with us, Joyce seemed to be doing much better. We were joking around, and I asked her, "Are you going to live with us forever and have me as your full-time nanny and cook?"

She was like, "Why would I pass that up?"

We both knew this arrangement was coming to an end. On Thursday of that week, I told her that maybe on Sunday we could move her back to her house. She looked at me, kind of jokingly, and kind of seriously: "You mean you don't want to take care of me forever?"

I just laughed because we both knew I'd reached my limit.

They moved back to their house that Sunday, and the Bible-study women started making food to send over to Joyce's house every day. I delivered that food at least three to four times a week for more than a year. At one point, Joyce said the meals were piling up in her fridge, so we cut back to only delivering every other day. Again, this was "church ladies" at their best. Not only did they make food, but they would send gifts sometimes for birthdays or Christmas. That May, they put on a beautiful birthday luncheon for Joyce at Carolyn's farmhouse.

I can picture her beaming on the deck that spring day, maybe the most beautiful I had ever seen her.

WEDDINGS
AND FUNERALS

Be thou the rainbow the storms of life.
The evening beam that smiles the clouds away,
and tints tomorrow with prophetic ray.

Lord Byron

Five days after Kara died, Teresa was a junior bridesmaid in a friend's wedding. She did great, walking the aisle in her beautiful dress we'd picked out at Nordstrom, lighting candles, and then returning to the pew to sit by me.

Suddenly, without any warning, Teresa broke down. She was sobbing uncontrollably in the church pew and eventually walked out of the sanctuary. She didn't fully tell me what was going on until much later in her life.

Sitting there, watching the ceremony, it hit her that I wouldn't be at her wedding. There was no part of her, and no part of me, that thought I would be alive to be the mother of the bride.

I'd had a similar experience a few years earlier on a long flight coming home from New Zealand. It was the middle of the night, and I was stuck in a long row of seats in the center of the plane watching a movie on a large screen several seats in front of me. The movie was *Father of the Bride*. It was a comedy, and I was really looking forward to seeing it. But, about an hour in, I was hysterically messy crying, gasping for breath crying, people staring at me kind of crying. I absolutely lost it for the exact same reason—the realization that I wouldn't be at my kids' weddings.

The truth was, always in our lives during those years of uncertainty, with death lingering at our door, we lived with an underlying awareness that our happiness now would not make up for our sadness later.

During the first years of HIV, I tried to keep everything on the outside seemingly normal and even happy, though on the inside I was thinking about death and dying all the time. I was constantly surrounded by death and people dying, and I thought I was managing to control what my kids knew and saw. I tried desperately to hide or shield them from the pain and sadness. I thought they were being protected by my constant focus on what was positive and by keeping our lives separated from my world of AIDS.

Kara dying changed all of that. Kara was a child, their friend. They had watched their friend die of AIDS. If I had been sheltering them from death, that shelter was shattered.

More than four hundred people showed up at Fourth Memorial Church on a beautiful fall day in Spokane to celebrate Kara's life. The remembrance, wrapped thoroughly in her personality, had been planned from her hospital bed before she died. At that point, she'd been to several funerals of our many friends on the speakers' bureau who'd died. Kara understood, even as a seven-year-old, what a person would include in a memorial service.

One of her requests was that there would be twelve songs in the program sung and led by various people she'd chosen: her mom, her brothers, and her Grandma Joyce. The church was filled to capacity. It was a long service but also alive, with plenty of laughter mixed with tears.

Being that it had been more than a month since Kara died, a death everyone saw coming, I think people already had processed a bit, which allowed this remembrance to be more upbeat than most funerals I've been to. It was impossible to keep a serious atmosphere with so many small children in the room, running around in their Sunday-best outfits, singing Kara's many songs, and even telling stories about their sweet friend.

I don't remember all twelve of the songs that Kara picked to sing, but I do remember that we sang "This little light of mine, I'm gonna let it shine," because the next day, on October 8, Teresa and I had our picture on the front page of the *Spokesman Review* Sunday newspaper with our fingers in the air doing the hand motions.

In a quote from her pastor about those songs, he said, "You have to do the hand motions or Kara will be displeased … She wanted her brothers up here and me with the guitar and you looking silly. Those were her orders."

I asked Teresa what she remembered.

"I remember that day as a really fun day," she said.

I think Kara would have been very happy about that.

NEW YORK

London is satisfied, Paris is resigned,
but New York is always hopeful.
Always it believes that something good
is about to come off, and it must hurry to meet it.

Dorothy Parker

Right before Christmas in 1995, Scott and I flew to New York City for a fun romantic getaway. He'd given me the trip for my birthday the summer before. Since going public as a speaker and spending countless hours supporting our new community as well as battling illness myself, our lives had become a stressful blend of rushing between school events, soccer practices, recitals, and the intense world of AIDS, which this past year had included the loss of Kara and additional support for Joyce and her boys. Both of us were desperate for a break; we were spent. We needed to leave town to flee our real lives, in a way transforming into other people. Escaping our realities, we headed to the Big Apple, hoping to soak ourselves in pure fun.

Spokane Julie is the AIDS lady, a mother of three who's exhausted by nine o'clock every night. New York Julie goes to Broadway musicals and eats out for every meal. She's in the East Coast time zone and can stay awake past midnight.

I'd not been to New York City since high school when I lived there for three weeks with my dance troupe, and I'd never been there for the holidays—a sight to see, every block magically lit up.

Scott planned this excursion so far in advance that he managed to snag front-row seats at four big Broadway shows: *Les Misérables, Cats, Phantom of the Opera,* and *Beauty and the Beast.* I love musicals. Our whole family loves musicals.

While attending the shows, Scott and I were introduced to the nonprofit Broadway Cares/Equity Fights AIDS, which was raising funds at Broadway events for AIDS-related critical services in all fifty states, Puerto Rico, and Washington, D.C. I noticed on the list of recipients the AIDS network in Seattle where I first went when I was diagnosed. (By 2020 Broadway Cares/Equity Fights AIDS had given over three-hundred-million dollars to the effort to care for and support people living with HIV.)

The front row is indescribable on Broadway. Two scenes come to mind from our front-row experience, one good, one not so much. The first was having one of the cats, from *Cats,* grab candy from Scott's box of Dots and eat it right in front of us in the middle of the production—so fun! Front-row seats at their best.

The second memorable front-row experience was a full-on drama during *Phantom of the Opera.* As soon as the lights went down and the chandelier went up, I suddenly had the urge to throw up. These things happen when you have AIDS, and as much as I wanted to be staying up late in New York, taking a vacation from my regular life, taking a vacation from a disease is not so easy. So, there I was, in the front row and not at all close to the aisle, where no one can be up moving around after the show starts. Escape was not possible.

Unfortunately, New York Julie only carried the tiniest of clutches. I was desperately wishing for Spokane Julie's mom-purse which could easily have doubled as a barf bag.

The waves of nausea were causing me to perspire, and I was suddenly very aware that anything I did would be witnessed by an entire theater of people. I spent the performance focused on the orchestra pit, trying to decide where the best direction to puke would be. Trumpets looked easier to clean than cellos. Would I be the first person to puke into the orchestra pit at the Majestic Theater, or was this a semi-regular occurrence? If this was the first time, would this be notable enough to get a mention in the *New York Times* theater section? I was absolutely miserable, yet somehow, I held it together until intermission. As soon as the lights went up, I practically climbed over the elderly couple between me and the nearest exit.

This brings me to the heart of that whole trip and how, on one level, it was a complete disaster while also being the trip of a lifetime.

A few nights after arriving, we met up with some longtime friends, Dave and Teresa Hillis. They were in New York with their three boys on a family trip before going down to North Carolina for a larger family gathering. Dave's brother and his wife had lost their eight-year-old to a brain aneurysm the March before, and their extended family was having Christmas together in a special place, since it was the first without J.D. We went to college with Dave and Teresa, and never did we think that in our mid-thirties we would be burying children. Our conversation was dominated by that topic ... Kara and J.D. ... seven- and eight-year-olds.

Dave had a favorite restaurant by the Tavern on the Green in Central Park, so we decided to walk there and get dinner. Plowing through the snow for a couple of miles, we eventually found the place, and being super hungry we ordered all of the suggested specialties on the menu.

By the time the food came, my cold body had shivered its

way into starvation, so I gleefully warmed it up by gorging myself. That night, after returning to our hotel and then for the next several days, I embarked on being the sickest I had been in years. Just as I was almost feeling better, I would put something in my mouth, and it would come out both ends.

I ended up in the emergency room in New York City, which took a whole day of my life and, other than getting some fluids, wasn't a ton of help. The best thing I could do was not eat anything. I went to shows, I went to fancy dinners with Scott, and, at the most, I would have a tiny bit of water. I just didn't want to miss out on anything and not eating was the only solution allowing me to experience a little of what we had planned.

Dave's son, Patrick, would in future years marry our daughter, Teresa, and we would go on to be lifelong friends who shared grandkids. In those future years, I would refer to this night in New York City as "the night Dave tried to kill me at his favorite New York restaurant." But, despite being reminded by my battered intestines that I, indeed, had a compromised immune system, New York had been an oasis in the desert for us, a badly needed escape. As we landed in Spokane on Christmas Eve, I was grateful that we had the means to leave our world, if only for a few days.

And I was grateful to be home.

FIVE O'CLOCK CHARLIE

It is one of the blessings of old friends
that you can afford to be stupid with them.

Ralph Waldo Emerson

'm not sure I can accurately describe our neighborhood and the people we lived next to and hung out with in Spokane. I've told you about my neighbor Paula, the nurse who had the most chill response ever when I told her I was HIV-positive. Paula was married to John, and they lived in a cul-de-sac near our house. They had moved from their house to the house right next door because they loved our neighborhood but needed a bigger house for their growing family of four boys. Paula and John plus two other families in the neighborhood, some add-on friends, and Scott and I were part of a group of us that met for dinner every Sunday night most weeks of the year.

I'm not sure when this "dinner group" started, but we weren't in the initial crew. The dinner would rotate between our houses and was called "5 o'clock Charlie." Whoever could make it would convene at five o'clock on Sunday, and this happened for years. We participated in 5 o'clock Charlie every Sunday that we could for ten years, and it had been happening before us and went on after we moved.

John had been in the Air Force and was a big fan of the TV show *MASH*. The name 5 o'clock Charlie came from the episode where every afternoon, at five, a North Korean pilot would fly overhead and let loose a bomb, attempting to hit the hospital dump. The pilot, nicknamed "5 o'clock Charlie," was so reliably unsuccessful that the officers in the 4077th began a daily betting pool based on how far away from the target his bomb would land. Since our dinner started at five, somehow this became its name.

5 o'clock Charlie had rules. If it didn't have rules, I don't think it would have lasted so many years. One of the rules: you were not supposed to go to the store. It was a potluck of sorts where you brought whatever was in your fridge or whatever you could cook out of the things you had on hand. We all broke the rules occasionally, but, bottom line, your food couldn't be fancy or difficult—unless, of course, you were serving fancy dinner-party leftovers.

We rotated houses each week, so the pressure wasn't on any one family to host, and dinner varied greatly from week to week. One week, we'd be eating in a neighbor's backyard, the next, plopped in front of someone else's TV watching a Seahawks game or gathered around an outside fire pit set up in a neighbor's driveway. I might have brought leftovers from a taco dinner that would be paired with macaroni and cheese and a thrown-together salad. The point was to be there at five and spend more thought on the conversation and being together than on the food we were ingesting for dinner.

These neighbors—Paula and John, Pete and Jackie, and Bud and Di—became close friends and surrogate relatives on holidays. We celebrated birthdays and special occasions together, made crafts for Christmas in Di's craft room, and watched TV together on Thursdays back when the lineup was *Friends*, *Seinfeld*, and *E.R.* We even organized a huge party for the last episode of *Seinfeld*, a sad day for television.

One of our favorite neighborhood recipes was banana chocolate chip muffins, affectionately named "bombs." Many a Saturday morning, bombs would be delivered to our door by whoever had risen early with a surplus of brown bananas. To this day, occasionally one of my girls emails me and asks for "the bomb recipe." As I respond, I'm always wondering if the FBI will now be monitoring my online activity.

Looking back, I realize that we were incredibly lucky to be surrounded by amazing friends during those hard years. Our neighborhood felt like a place where we could be "normal," yet also a safe place to share hard things. If it sounds like we lived in a *Leave it to Beaver* or *Full House* TV set on Windsong Avenue in the 1990s, that wouldn't be far from the truth.

I'm not sure what we would have done without our neighbors during that era; they became a spring in a very dry time.

GEORGE

What friends or kindred can be so close
and intimate as the powers of our soul,
which, whether we will or not,
must ever bear us company?

Saint Teresa of Avila

When I first met George Cheney, he was barely over a hundred pounds, and I was thinking that he couldn't get any smaller. But this was AIDS; there were few of us who didn't get smaller. We were wasting away in some form or another, either from the disease or from the medications we were on.

Though he was little in stature, George was large in kindness and excelled in another thing I love—critical thinking. When I helped start the support group, I asked George what he thought about it, and he told me, "Be careful not to hurt people. Be kind. Be gentle."

It was the first of many times that George Cheney would give me wise advice.

We became fast friends for so many reasons. For all of our many differences, we had a number of things in our life that were similar, things we shared. George and I shared the same birthday, July 16. George and I are both the youngest in our families; we were raised Lutheran and had quite a history with religion and the church. The two of us both became teachers and valued education.

And if that wasn't enough in common, this is where it gets eerie. George attended seminary and became a Lutheran minister, randomly becoming the pastor of a church in a tiny Washington town called Endicott, the rural farm town I was born in. My family attended that very church long before he came to town. I was baptized in that little church. George and I could name several families in Endicott that we both knew.

When he told his church community, as well as the people he worked with as the chaplain at Eastern Washington University, that he had AIDS, it did not go well.

I listened to George speak about this several times. He would say, "Most of the people I have worked with—my colleagues, other ministers, and professionals—have stopped talking to me. They completely ignore me. These are people that I have known for years and years. I knew their families; I knew their problems and pains. I used to drink with them, cry with them, and laugh with them."

He never said this with anger; he was gracious, yet extremely sad.

From the beginning of our relationship, I knew that George's heart had been greatly affected by HIV and by the different medicines he had been given, not just medication for AIDS, but also chemotherapy. George used to tell me, "I'm going to die of a broken heart."

Looking back, I don't remember a time when George wasn't sick. He just kept going, so I never really imagined him dying. As his health began to fail, I would see him less and less often. I called and asked what he needed and made deliveries to his apartment. The apartment felt dark to me, depressing. Making those deliveries made me sad because it seemed George was becoming as depressed as the place in which he was living.

Nonetheless, George and I shared a lot of laughs. I've never put much thought or belief into the astrological signs, but we had very similar personalities, which made me wonder if being under the sign of Cancer might mean something. Was there a uniqueness to being born on the same day? Both of us liked being smart, we liked learning things, but most of all, we liked being in control. He was a genuine control freak like me.

I hadn't seen George in quite a while, but I heard he was in the hospital and that he was not taking visitors. And then I got a call. It was George, and he said, "I don't have much longer and there are only a few people that I'm letting visit. I want you to come; I want to see you."

His heart was ready to give out, and it would not last through the week. As he had predicted, he was literally dying of a broken heart.

This was the only time in my life I remember talking to someone knowing full well that I would never talk to them again. It felt unreal because George seemed very coherent, and yet he was going to have heart failure soon.

I was trying hard not to be depressing and drag on about how much I was going to miss him; he already knew that. I tried to tell George what he had meant to me but I'm so bad at sharing seriously sad things without bursting into tears. At best, it was a feeble effort.

The one thing I remember saying to George was how weird it was going to be that someday I might be older than him on our birthday. I said, "I guess on that day you can have the last laugh because you will forever be younger and hotter than I am."

He laughed. I smiled.

I never saw George alive again.

Several weeks later, I went to his memorial service. The big surprise came in the middle of his memorial service when it was time for someone to give a homily or sermon. All of a sudden, over the speaker, loud and clear was George's voice. He had recorded his own sermon for his memorial.

All I could think was, "Oh my gosh, way to play the final card, George!" He got the last word, even in death.

THE QUILT

The song ended but the melody lingers on.

Irving Berlin

At the beginning of 1996, we heard that the Names Project AIDS Memorial Quilt would be coming to the Spokane Convention Center. At that time many people who died of AIDS did not have funerals, due to both the stigma of AIDS and the refusal by many funeral homes and cemeteries to handle the deceased's remains. Sewing a panel for the Quilt was often the only opportunity survivors had to remember and celebrate their loved ones' lives.

That April, Spokane was hosting 920 3-foot-by-6-foot quilt panels and was expecting around 8000 people to view the display. At that time, it consisted of 32,000 panels, each bundled by region, city, and zip code, so the panels from Washington State had been requested.

Scott and I decided it would be a meaningful experience for our whole family if we volunteered at the Quilt. Joyce and the boys planned to volunteer, as Kara's new quilt panel was to be dedicated and they had never seen Joyce's husband's panel sewn into the larger quilt squares. Debbie, being a quilter, made Carolyn's brother, Chuck, a panel that was also going to be dedicated.

Joyce, Debbie, Scott, and I attended three workshops to learn our roles, the history of the Quilt, how to unfold the large square sections during the opening ceremony, and how to refold it during the closing ceremony. People could sign up to read names because, at all times while the Quilt was being displayed, names of those who had lost their lives would be read from a podium.

The final workshop, on-site at the convention center, began after the semitrucks containing the Quilt had arrived. Because the kids were participating in the ceremonies, they all came to this last volunteer session. We helped place quilt pieces, and we all practiced the opening and closing ceremonies. At the time it seemed like fun and, even though we could see and read all of the panels, the reality of their impact had not yet set in.

We learned in our workshop that volunteers needed to wear white and not have shoes on, both to keep the Quilt clean and to honor and respect those who had died. So, on Saturday, April 27, dressed in white clothes from head to toe, the five of us headed to the convention center to participate in the Quilt ceremony.

The kids were in jovial spirits, not only because they had the privilege to participate in this exciting community event but also because they would spend the day with the Claypool boys. On the way there, everyone was making fun of Scott's all-white dress shirt and shorts, saying that he looked like he should be driving an ice cream truck and laughingly calling him the "Ice Cream Man."

The emotional response that descended on all of us came as a bit of a surprise because the day had been so lighthearted and even fun-filled. When we got to the convention center, all of the loud activities and busyness of setting up the display the night before were replaced by a quiet somber presence, similar to what you would experience walking into a funeral home. The opening ceremony felt deep and important, and the kids performed their parts unfolding the quilt with a seriousness that made me proud and teary-eyed.

When the ceremony finished, the viewing of the Quilt opened to the general public. People who'd been watching us were free to roam around on walkways between the large quilt squares and view the panels. I looked up to see that all our neighbors from our weekly "5 o'clock Charlie" dinner group were there with tears in their eyes, visibly touched by the whole thing.

As I walked around, out of the corner of my eye I saw my neighbor and friend, Di, hunched down over a small person with her arms around them. I looked closer and there was Laura, sobbing uncontrollably while looking at Joyce's husband's quilt. Di knelt down next to her holding her tightly. My heart broke watching her.

Laura had talked about AIDS the least, avoiding the topic most times it came up.

I realized in that moment that she harbored a storehouse of thoughts, worries, and fears, brewing inside her; on this day, they were finally spilling out. I loved Di in that moment as one of my most treasured and precious friends. I think she had always felt a special way for Laura and showed up with a mountain of comfort in a way that my daughter desperately needed.

Many tears were shed that weekend as Kara's quilt panel was dedicated and names of people we knew who had lost the fight were read out loud. I am sure my children will never forget that weekend. Ryan recently told me that, other than Kara dying, the Quilt experience was one of his most vivid memories.

It was a visual reminder that no matter how positive we were spinning this life with AIDS, people who were infected often died.

The next fall, the entire AIDS Quilt was displayed on the National Mall in Washington, D.C. At that time, it covered thirteen acres or twelve football fields. The Quilt had grown to 39,000 panels and they were expecting up to 5,000 more to be dedicated during the event. An estimated 750,000 people came to view it during the three-day event, including the Presidential Democratic Nominee, Bill Clinton, and his wife, Hillary Rodham Clinton. That was the last time the whole quilt was exhibited because it grew too large for any venue or outdoor space to display it.

Pat, Debbie, and all three of their kids went to Washington, D.C., along with Carolyn and Ed, who took Craig. They saw Carolyn's brother's quilt and Kara's, both now sewn into the bigger quilt. They marched with thousands of people in a candlelight vigil from the Capitol to the Lincoln Memorial. One of the days, Carolyn read names at the podium on the Mall, including her brother, Chuck's.

To this day, one of my biggest regrets is that I didn't go. I could have gone, but for reasons I cannot remember, I decided to stay home.

DEATH IS COMPLICATED

It is not death that a man should fear,
but he should fear never beginning to live.

Marcus Aurelius

During these years in Spokane, death became a frequent visitor. In our first year, I got a call from Chris that Harold, one of his best friends who was also dear to our family, had died of AIDS. Mary, from camp, and then this friend, Harold, were the first people I knew personally who died of AIDS, but they were the beginning of a long train that brought sadness to our small community.

Our speakers' bureau had a wide variety of personalities and characters. I've told you about Mark and some of the things he would talk about when speaking to groups, how he always felt like his message was resonating with someone in the audience even though people were often uncomfortable with his stories of addiction and abuse. I loved that he always had an opinion and lived his life out loud, wearing every emotion on his sleeve.

Mark, the life of every party, was an artist. He was extravagant and full of interesting news. Mark's partner, Tony, wasn't infected with HIV but suffered from serious liver disease. Tony was the perfect calm to Mark's drama.

Mark and Tony came to most things the speakers' bureau took part in and were often on panels speaking with me. As outgoing and upbeat as Mark was, his story was actually very sad. I could say this about several speakers but, in particular, Mark. His story left me feeling like most of his jovial personality was masking some very dark events in his life. Kids, especially high school and college kids, loved to hear him speak and related to what he had to say.

Well, two facts about Mark ... first of all, he was a hairstylist and cut my hair. Secondly, he had an infection called cytomegalovirus, which was causing him to go blind. It was the same virus that caused Craig to go blind—a virus that didn't affect healthy people but created catastrophe for a person with AIDS.

This means that for a while I had a blind person cutting my hair. And I wasn't the only one; other friends were also getting haircuts from him. We would have these discussions on the sly about how long we could let this go on. How blind would we let Mark get, subjecting our locks to his scissors?

Mark was an artist; this is what he did. The thought that he couldn't do it anymore broke our hearts. So we kept going. I remember telling him the last few times, "Not too much, Mark, just a trim! Just a little bit off the ends." I was amazed at how many times my hair looked pretty good despite it all—though occasionally I had to find someone else to even it out.

Mark and Tony also owned a quilt shop. Another thing that required eyesight. It was sad to hear him talk about going blind.

"It's not fun to sit here and watch my eyesight go," he'd say. "Half of the stuff I used to do I can't do anymore. I'm a magazine reader. I subscribe to tons of magazines; I can't read them anymore. I'm starting my braille classes because, if this is going to continue and I go blind, I would prefer to have braille right now so I can see what I'm doing instead of waiting until I'm completely blind."

I am not sure when, but at one point Mark and Tony moved out of state to be with family. We never expected it, but Tony died before Mark, and soon after Mark joined him. After he died, I was given a little film vial and told that part of Mark's ashes were in it. He wanted everyone he knew to spread his ashes in a special place to remember him. I had that vial on my desk at work for over a year.

I would stare at it and think to myself, "Okay, Mark, where should I put you?"

Eventually, I took the vial home and spread Mark's ashes under my butterfly bush in my backyard. As I sprinkled, I whispered, "Fly away, dear one." I imagined a big, gaudy, beautiful, and sparkly butterfly rising up into the blue sky.

I still think of Mark and all of the living he packed into his life. He left an impression that lingers and still makes me smile.

The last time I saw Barry, I was walking down the street in downtown Spokane and Barry happened to be driving the other way in his truck. It was a warm day, and his windows were down. He yelled at me to get my attention, "Hey, Julie!" and then with a huge smile, he waved at me.

I said, "Hey! You look good!" loud enough for him to hear and waved back.

I love that image of Barry in his truck, wind in his hair, full of motion and energy. He was a deep well, a beautiful and complicated soul.

Not long after, I heard Barry had died. It was sudden and devastating news; I hope he finally found the peace he deserved.

Harold, Mark, and Barry were all artists, as were many of our friends who died. So much was lost when all these friends died. They were a wealth of beauty and goodness, creativity and humor. I wonder: what would these artists have created?

What void was left that might have been filled with their imaginations and creativity?

These were not "old" people. They were young and often in the prime of their lives. Without disclosing any personal information, it's important to note that not everyone who had HIV died of complications from AIDS. Some opted for a faster route and chose their own time; others had multiple health complications making it hard to assess what the actual cause of death was.

Some deaths stung worse than others and none felt more like a tragedy than Camie's.

Camie had moved back to Montana because as she became sick and was hospitalized, she had no one to take care of her son. It made sense to go home where she had more support. Knowing she was going to die, she wanted her little guy to bond with the greater family who would take care of him.

On Easter Sunday, the 30th of March in 1997, I got a call from Camie's brother saying that she had died. She was thirty-four years old. Her brother thanked me for being her friend and asked me if there was anything they could do with the box full of medicine that was left over; was there anyone who could use it? I told him to mail it to me and that I would pass it on to AID FOR AIDS in New York City, who recycled AIDS meds by sending them to other countries where there were shortages. It was and still is illegal to redistribute them in the US.

I was so sad to hear Camie had died, but I wasn't surprised. She'd made it far longer than I thought she would. The last conversation I had with her still makes me laugh. She was telling me that in her support group, in Montana, everyone was a cowboy ... so many boots, hats, and giant buckles.

I said, "Why don't you find the gay men's support group and join that?"

She paused and laughed, "Julie ... that *is* the gay support group!"

I still smile when I think of it. Of course the gay men would be cowboys in Montana. What was I thinking?

After my core group of friends began to die, I started to hold back on new relationships with people who were infected. It was hard to meet someone new and set myself up once more to possibly lose them. I began to have new boundaries to protect myself from future losses that, emotionally, I wasn't able to handle.

I also didn't want my friends to seem replaceable. Some piece of me saw new relationships as replacements, somehow taking away from the meaningful ones I had lost and, in my grieving mind, lessening the memory of those friends. I wanted to keep their memories and spirits alive as much as possible, for as long as possible. I dove into a serious grieving process, becoming fairly unavailable to strangers. I guess in some way, I didn't want to be replaceable. I didn't want people to forget me and move on quickly when I died. The bottom line is death is complicated. There are no formulas.

I don't think I realized at the time just how special it was to be living in Spokane in the 1990s, as a person infected with HIV. Spokane was a city that was just big enough to have some things: we had a few of the amenities of a big city, like opera, and we were big enough that Broadway musicals would come on tour; we had a minor-league baseball team. When it came to HIV, Spokane had an AIDS network, there were comprehensive care services, and we had access to several physicians who specialized in HIV. But, it wasn't Seattle. In Seattle, the HIV community services included long-term survivor groups, men's groups, and a group that focused on women. The beauty of Spokane was that we weren't that big, so for most of the 1990s there was basically one group: people who were infected with HIV and living with AIDS. We were a very diverse group of people all mixed together and I, for one, really liked that.

I did, in those years, crave the possibility of having a women's group for HIV, and for a while, we tried to get one going. At the time, I thought it would be ideal. When that became a reality for me, I just missed the guys so much and realized what a blessing it had been to be in a town where AIDS was not segregated according to any kind of classification. It was just a bunch of people who were dumped together in the most magical, comical, and tragic way.

That I might not have ever known George, or Craig, or Barry, or Mark and Tony is unthinkable.

THE QUESTION

Hope is the thing with feathers
that perches in the soul—
and sings the tunes without the words—
and never stops at all.

Emily Dickinson

The summer of 1998 was, again, filled with camps. We returned to the camp in Canada for another month; our kids were getting older and, at that point, had spent almost ten summers of their lives at camp. The girls were helpful to the staff and kept busy scooping ice cream in the snack bar. Ryan spent a ton of time with the musicians who played songs at most of the camp's large meetings. He was becoming very proficient on guitar, and it was clear he had a "thing" for music.

That summer I turned forty! I know many people hit the big 4-0 and grieve the loss of their youth, but for me, it truly was a celebration. This was one of the many milestones I never thought I'd reach in the early days of my diagnosis. Scott threw me a surprise party hosted by some good friends. What I noticed most when looking back at the photos was that none of my friends with HIV, including Joyce, were invited. People from my Bible study, the neighbors, some work friends, and, of course, Debbie and Pat were there. As I looked at the photos it was a stark reminder that I was still living my life in buckets—I separated people into categories and almost never mixed them together. It makes me feel sad and disappointed in myself to reflect on this, but it's hard to deny the truth when it is recorded on film in front of you.

I guess I separated things to simplify. I would also say that bringing the Claypool boys into our lives, up to our lake cabin, and on overnights at our house was the beginning of breaking down those neat little compartments. It was the beginning of mixing all kinds of people together in a beautiful and somewhat messy existence.

We'd cared for the Claypool boys often since Kara died, especially Dale. As Joyce's health began failing, conversations arose about what might happen to her boys if she died. At first, she was in huge denial that she needed to set up a place for them to go. She would say, "If I just hang on long enough, they will be old enough to stay here in our house and live on their own." Being that she'd been in the Marines, she began preparing them with "life skills" to survive. When I asked Dale, he also was convinced that should his mom die, he could just stay in their house and live with his brother, on their own.

Late that summer was the first time Joyce asked me if Scott and I would consider taking Dale into our home after she died. At the time she'd already made arrangements for Chris to live in the Spokane Valley where several family "homes" allowed kids to be paired with guardians and live in a structured community. I never questioned Joyce's decision to separate the boys; she knew their individual needs and was doing her best to set them up to succeed after she was gone.

I said I would talk to Scott and think about it. It was a question we had thought about even before she asked. We'd been taking Dale along on some of our family outings and adventures since he was in fifth grade, and now he was starting his first year of high school. The thing was, the question was no longer hypothetical. Joyce was going to die. Dale and Chris would not be allowed to stay alone and raise themselves. They were still too young at twelve and fourteen.

It was a lot to think about, but I had a sense, deep down, as did Scott, that we knew the answer.

WHITE CHRISTMAS

May your days be merry and bright.
And may all your Christmases be white.

Irving Berlin

In the fall, Joyce's health began to go downhill. She was always fragile, but she began to have high fevers that wouldn't go away and infections the doctors could not get on top of. On World AIDS Day, December 1, Joyce gave a speech at the University of Idaho in an auditorium filled with students. Little did we know, in twenty-three days, she would be gone.

That December, I still brought food to the Claypools' house a couple of times a week. One day, I stopped by, and Joyce was lying on her couch; she was sweating, obviously running a high fever. She told me she needed to drive Dale to hockey.

"I can take him," I said.

She looked up, smiled, and replied, "I might as well die at hockey as die here on this couch." She was not joking.

At the beginning of the month, all Joyce talked about was Christmas. She loved singing and was constantly humming or belting out Christmas carols. She looked weak, with dark circles under her eyes; those circles betrayed the smile on her face and her positive attitude. I began to know deep in my gut that she was near the end.

Like many of our friends who succumbed to the virus, Joyce was having a hard time keeping food down and had been put on a bland diet. One day when the boys were at school, she began pleading with me to take her to Bruchi's, a fast-food place that made killer cheesesteaks.

"No," I kept saying back. "That is not a good idea."

"Come on. I might never get to have one again," she whined with sad puppy eyes. I wish I could say that her efforts were not effective, but I eventually gave in.

It took a long time to get her in street clothes and into my car. She was walking slowly at the mall, but we managed to make it to the food court. Once at our table, I said I would order but she insisted she wanted to get her own and proceeded to ask for a whole, huge, chicken cheesesteak. I interrupted and told the server that they needed to cut it in half so we could share and could they please put on a fraction of the usual amount of onions.

At that moment, I seriously felt like I was her mom, not her friend. I was pretty sure this outing was a huge mistake that I would regret. It was like watching my toddler eat their third piece of cake knowing they'd probably be crazy on a sugar-high, or sick to their stomach, in a couple of hours. But the pure happiness and joy on her face made me smile. Like Camie's last big meal, I never saw Joyce eat anything like that again.

Joyce was admitted to the hospital about three weeks before Christmas. At the time, I was busy with my seasonal job at a department store downtown, overloaded with speaking engagements, and juggling all of the holiday shopping. I went to visit her as much as I could on my way to work and even snuck in a few times in the wee hours after my shift. There were always a ton of people hanging out in her room, so we didn't have many private conversations. A mutual friend was her hospice nurse and was almost always with Joyce.

One day I stopped by, and Joyce had half the nursing staff as an audience while singing "White Christmas" to them. "White Christmas" was her favorite. At that point Joyce had almost completely lost her hearing; to say she had become tone-deaf would be an understatement. Yet there she was, singing at the top of her lungs, maybe hoping she could hear herself. Everyone in the room ended up belting it out with her; Joyce had that effect on people.

One night when it was just the two of us, she asked me, again, if Scott and I would take Dale, at least until he graduated high school. She had broached this topic several times, but I'd never given an answer. It wasn't until that night, in the hospital, I said yes. Of course, Scott and I had discussed the possibility for some time and had agreed that we would do this, but I was alone with her when I said yes. She cried, sobbed actually, and hugged me tight. It was the last time I was alone with Joyce.

Joyce hung on longer than anyone predicted. Her greatest joy every day, besides seeing her boys, was getting wheeled to an outside space to have her cigarette. Being December, it was freezing, but somehow she managed. She didn't seem to mind the cold and loved the snow. My guess is that she had a raging fever most of the time and maybe the chill felt good to her.

Joyce died on December 23. She was thirty-five years old. I'd seen her a couple of days before and said to her face that she did not get to die on Christmas Eve or Christmas Day, so as to ruin those days for the rest of us forever. I had no idea it would be so close.

I was at work in the early evening of the twenty-third and noticed that Scott had left me a message. All he said was that I should call him right away.

When I called back, he said, "Joyce died, and they are waiting for you to come and see her ... if you want to."

All I said was, "Of course."

The instant I left work to go say my last goodbyes, at the very second I stepped outside, the church bells that played music every hour on the hour downtown began to toll their version of "White Christmas" and simultaneously it began to snow. Joyce's favorite Christmas carol was ringing out in the bells of our city. It was as if the bells were ringing because an angel had truly just gotten her wings.

This was a God moment. One of those rare times when I could sense the divine close to me. Where the space between heaven and earth seemed to thin, like there was just a slight shadow between here and there. I smiled and cried at the same time because I knew at that moment that Joyce had arrived where she most wanted to go.

As quirky as Joyce often was, I can't think of many people I would rather be dying with; she almost made it fun. She was my opposite in many ways, never overanalyzing life. After she died, I kept calling her answering machine to hear her voice and her cheery greeting.

Whether people admired her or disagreed with her methods, one thing was for sure, Joyce Claypool had captivated Spokane. She had put her whole life story out there for good or bad. She'd risked the well-being and the reputation of herself and her children. She made AIDS human to a whole community. Some would say she liked being in the spotlight for her own self-gratification; others thought she was a true saint who had sacrificed everything to keep others healthy.

All I know is, she was my friend. As with so many of us, there were layers of secrets, abuse, and hardship. But Joyce chose to use those to help others, like myself, have an easier time living with a disease that frightened most people. She was a person who loved easily, freely, and lavishly. It was probably her greatest quality and her biggest curse. She didn't hold resentments. She forgave easily. I never once heard Joyce Claypool say something bad about her husband, the man who was responsible for her death and the death of her child.

I think of her often, and I wonder what she would've done if she had lived twenty-five more years. I'm positive it would have been loud and purposeful.

PICKING UP THE PIECES

Grief never ends ... But it changes.
It's a passage, not a place to stay.
Grief is not a sign of weakness, nor lack of faith ...
It is the price of love.

Unknown Author

The day after Joyce died was Christmas Eve. I worked at the store until early afternoon and then came home to go to church and engage in our usual Christmas Eve rituals, playing our traditional present game and sharing our highs and lows from the year. My emotions were a roller coaster, and yet there was always a calming factor when the five of us were together. Having our solid traditions made it seem like there was still some sort of order in the world.

It did occur to me that our momentary calm could dissolve soon because we had just told a dying woman that her son could join our family. I was a bit unsettled thinking we were about to disrupt this great thing we had going with our original family of five by adding a new teenager to the mix. I reminded myself that I still believed that God was in control, and I felt that bringing Dale into our home was the right thing to do.

On Christmas Day we meandered across town to the Claypool house to hug the boys and bring gifts. Several relatives roamed around the house and made themselves at home on the couch. Both Dale and Chris seemed to be in good spirits. We invited them to come with us at the end of the week to our lake place for New Year's Eve, and someone approved. The rest of the week for me was a blur; there are a ton of photos from the New Year's Priest Lake celebration, which is the only way I'm sure it happened.

Because we had no legal guardianship pre-arranged, decisions for Dale and Chris were being made by their paternal grandmother and she had resolved that a couple in Joyce's church, who were foster parents, would take the boys until other legal guardianship was approved by the court.

Dale would joke that he now had to go back to middle school, every kid's nightmare. He'd been a ninth grader at Shadle Park High School, but at his new residence in the Spokane Valley, ninth grade was in middle school. I was kind of glad because Chris was in seventh grade, and this would at least ensure that the two of them were in the same school during the transition.

Our family spent time with Dale during the winter and spring after Joyce died, but he did not live at our house. We included him in most family functions, including birthdays, and he traveled with Scott to a ski camp. The proceedings to be his legal guardians were in motion, but our court date turned out to be well into the summer.

Dale turned fifteen in early summer and our neighborhood threw a party for him. We also began another remodel of our house, adding an extra bedroom in our basement so Teresa and Laura could both be downstairs. Dale would be upstairs in a room next to Ryan's. To transform the upstairs into a guy space we changed all the tile in the bathroom from pink to navy blue. Dale picked out paint colors for his room and Scott painted it before he moved in.

That summer flew by; we spent extensive time at our lake

place because construction workers occupied the house. The kids seemed "all in" on this plan to have Dale join our family. I was surprised to discover that I found four kids easier than three. With three you always had an odd person out, but with four it seemed you could divide up every which way—older kids, younger kids, or boys and girls—and everyone had a partner.

We finally had our day in court at the end of July. I got a little worried when the judge started by asking a very good question, "Is it a good idea to place Dale with another adult who could die of AIDS?"

I assured him that I was in fairly good health and, really, Dale would be on his own in three years when he graduated high school and turned eighteen. I never considered we might be rejected. In the end, the judge gave in and signed the guardianship agreement while we all breathed a sigh of relief.

Right after our court date, Dale moved into our house. It was early August, and he was excited to start football practice at what would be his new school, Ferris High School. Dale and Teresa, both sophomores, went on a houseboat trip on Lake Roosevelt right before school started. Teresa's friends became Dale's friends, and because we now had a girl and boy in the same grade, our house was a popular place for their friends to hang out.

When Dale started going to the high school by our house, from day one he told all of the teachers we were his mom and dad. He never mentioned Joyce or his dad. He never talked about the amount of loss he had already experienced at fifteen years old. I think Dale needed a break from it all, a time to feel like all the other kids.

I've learned over the years that when something feels wrong, listen more carefully to that inner voice and act on it.

Dale calling us his parents felt off, but I let it go. I wish I had stopped him for a moment and said, "Dale, just call us Scott and Julie. No one can replace your mom and dad."

I think it would've been a three-minute conversation that would have made complete sense to him, but that conversation never happened.

As parents, what we didn't account for fully was the trauma we all had endured. We didn't seek enough counsel in this area from specialists who deal with childhood trauma. We didn't insist on counseling for any of us, including Dale.

I've often criticized people who relish quick fixes, but it was me craving a quick fix this time. So, I understood when Dale said he didn't want to go to a counselor. I will admit now, I related to his fear that opening those experiences of loss to discussion would just continue the pain. To be honest, I didn't want to go to counseling either.

I thought to myself, "We can bring up counseling at a later date."

Many times, I have thought back to our decision to bring Dale into our family for those few years. In a way, we also said "yes" to interacting with and caring about his brother, his grandparents, and his extended family.

People have asked me, "Would you do it again?"

I'm not sure what all of the details were behind Joyce's decision when she asked us to take Dale into our home. As I reflect on our choice, I wish I had asked, "Why us? Why did you pick us?" It's something I have wondered about many times.

But ... would we say yes again?

When I put myself back in time at the side of Joyce's hospital bed with her asking me to help raise her son, every time I think back, no matter how I replay it, my response is always the same: Yes.

THE DAWN
OF A NEW ERA

Hope is a waking dream.

Aristotle

I spent the 1990s fighting to live and assuming I wouldn't make it to see the new millennium. When it came, with all of its Y2K confusion set to the soundtrack of Prince's "1999," I was happy to be there for all the hubbub.

There was a broad spectrum of what it looked like to anticipate the year 2000. On one end, there were the preppers. They were stockpiling food, water, and even guns, waiting for all hell to break loose when computer systems failed. We were given an audiobook entitled *Y2K: What Every Christian Should Know.* I'm slightly embarrassed to admit that I listened to it.

On the other end of the spectrum were those going all out to greet the new millennium in style, as if pretending to be rich and famous at the stroke of midnight would guarantee you a fancy life in the new millennium. Preparing for this included shopping for glittery dresses and finding the perfect party to attend.

I was decidedly somewhere in the middle of this and instead of spending our savings on bomb shelters or designer dresses, we rang in the year 2000 with our neighborhood 5 o'clock Charlie group. Our party wasn't a glamorous rave—it was better. I was surrounded by family and friends for this momentous event, firmly on the other side of my three-to-five-year prognosis.

Even as I looked to the future, the question of death still lingered. Yes, I'd made it to the new millennium, but some of my closest friends hadn't, and it was sobering to see it through that lens. I was grateful to be alive, but the idea that I was always just an illness or two away from death still haunted me and my family.

Teresa and Dale both turned sixteen in the year 2000, and with that, I got to experience the joyful terror of teaching my kids to drive. I was looking forward to their high school graduation, and we were beginning to talk about colleges, but I still wasn't expecting to be at any of my kids' weddings, and I know they weren't expecting me to be there either.

I didn't wake up one day, look at the date and say, "Oh gee, I'm still here, time to do some more living!" This was a continuation of the journey I'd been on since that day ten years prior when my life changed forever with an HIV diagnosis. That diagnosis was as if I'd been fired from my previous life. Survival became my full-time job. First, I was working to come to terms with this new reality and working to handle my meds, then working against the clock to make lasting memories with my kids. The desire to get back to what I was passionate about came gradually, sheerly through continuing to live.

Since I was a child, I'd had a passion for school, learning, and educating others. For the past ten years, purely for survival, I'd put a lot of that on hold. Through the speakers' bureau, I'd gotten a little bit of learning and educating, but I wanted more, and opportunities continued to come in small steps that I could fit into my life, amidst being a mom, wife, and managing my disease.

The first big step had been back in the fall of 1998 when I went back to school. I enrolled at Eastern Washington University to renew my teaching certificate and add a health endorsement, hoping to go to work in public health. I took four classes, exactly the number of credits I needed for the certificate.

Eastern was a good forty-minute jaunt from our house, and my first class started at eight. Mornings came early and were busy, especially as the autumn days continued to grow colder and darker. I would get myself together, make sure the kids were getting ready for school, make lunches, and try to be out the door at quarter after seven, JanSport backpack full of coursework and my midday HIV meds.

Taking on school was rough. My morning handful of medications didn't stay down if I didn't eat enough. These meds were released over several hours; the minute my stomach became empty, up they'd come. More than one day was spent sitting in class, trying to pay attention while simultaneously gagging if I needed to run out and puke. Nevertheless, I made it through, achieving a renewed teaching certificate with an added health endorsement.

I'd spent the 1990s coming to terms with how delicate and uncertain life could be. No matter how solid we feel, one little thing can bring our world crashing down, and, whether we like it or not, we have to keep going. It's not possible to suddenly become a new and better person at the stroke of midnight, but if one keeps plowing forward, sometimes with the current, sometimes against it, what feels like an insurmountable task one day, might become possible in the future. When I first began taking antiretrovirals in 1990, it was a struggle to get dressed and make it out of the house, yet here I was ten years later, looking for a way to meaningfully rejoin the workforce.

The potential Y2K disaster was a lot of hype. So much went into preparing for a catastrophe that never happened, when in actuality, we were hit with a real disaster no one expected the following year, on September 11. We watched the disaster unfold on TV before the kids left for school. This is how life is: we prepare for one disaster, and then, when no one is looking, another one happens, yet again reminding us that life isn't ever as certain as one thinks.

DISCLOSURE

It's never too late to give up our prejudices.

Henry David Thoreau

'd heard that there was a sudden opening for a seventh-grade science teacher at one of the area middle schools because one of the teachers had to quit the second week of school. I was a Washington State certified biology and earth science teacher and now, since going back to school, I'd also added a health educator endorsement.

I knew I was qualified to teach seventh-grade science because the curriculum is basically a combination of earth and life sciences. Insider information, from someone at the school, was that they had no other applicants with science education experience. I was the most qualified person who applied for this job. Even if they added other kinds of science to their curriculum, I'd also taught physics and chemistry at the high school level.

With my three years of science teaching experience, both in high school and at the middle school level, I figured I had a good chance of getting this position. I decided to apply for the job.

The school district ended up hiring a first-year PE teacher to teach seventh-grade science with no science teaching background or experience. Was I overlooked and passed by for this job because I had AIDS and had been very public about my disease? It seemed pretty obvious.

People have their own ideas of what it might be like to have HIV, and they act according to those beliefs. I've told Scott many times that if he was ever infected with HIV, we should tell no one. The last thing Scott needed in furthering his career would be for people to think or know he had HIV. The reality of possibly being passed over for promotions, being purposely overlooked because people had assumptions about his health, wasn't something I wanted him to experience.

I am reminded of all the legitimate reasons why some people choose not to disclose their HIV status. I know a few of those people. One man Scott worked with recently has been infected since the early 1980s and has told only a handful of people.

An infected person might have a harder time getting a job. Not only might an employer look at HIV as somewhat of a liability, just for the increased price of their health insurance policy, which might increase premiums for the whole office, but also, the employer might assume that a person with HIV is going to be sick often and not be able to come to work. There are laws that protect people once they're in the workplace. The Americans with Disabilities Act of 1990 says businesses can't discriminate and need to accommodate anyone with HIV. The easiest way around accommodating would be to never hire that person in the first place.

There are many other reasons not to disclose that you're HIV-positive. I've heard people share about being rejected or judged by family and friends or about being shut out of their community at large when they find out about an AIDS diagnosis. Some of these stories are heartbreaking, and many include having to disclose one's sexual orientation at the same time. It's complicated and sometimes people just don't want to go there.

HIV is different from other groups of people who are discriminated against because many of us don't necessarily look sick and can hide it. We can lie, like I did for four years when I was first diagnosed.

There are also situations where choosing not to disclose HIV status is almost impossible. One of those is needing major medical help, like surgery. In the fall of 2000, I needed an emergency appendectomy and was told I needed to be operated on as soon as possible. Unfortunately, "as soon as possible" ended up being many hours later after my appendix had ruptured because the hospital couldn't find a surgeon willing to operate on an HIV-positive person.

This wasn't 1990; it was ten years later. I was in shock that this kind of fear was still happening. In reality, my experience would have been so different if I had needed this surgery before I was diagnosed, in the years I was infected with HIV and didn't know it. Those surgeons would have just used universal precautions and treated me like anyone else. Having to disclose that I was HIV-positive opened me up to fear and prejudice that has the possibility of being deadly in a medical setting.

The bottom line is, there are still reasons, good reasons, to not disclose that one is HIV-positive, and I respect anyone who chooses to keep their HIV status private.

EDUCATION
AND ADVOCACY

Start by doing what is necessary;
then do what is possible;
and suddenly you are doing the impossible.

Saint Francis of Assisi

"It's always fun to share your sex life with a classroom of
sixteen-year-olds!" said no one ever. Yes, an experience
others would probably rank up there on the list of most
awkward nightmares was a recurring daytime activity for me
as a part of the speakers' bureau.

One of the questions always asked by kids when I was
doing HIV education, especially high school students, was,
"Can you still have sex with your husband?"

And that was usually followed by, "And do you?"

Followed by, "I mean, does he still want to?"

Or, "Is he afraid of you?"

Kids ask the darndest things, don't they?

One time after asking this question a student added,
"Inquiring minds want to know."

This cracked me up. I mean, all of the adults wanted to
know these things too, but rarely would they ask.

Sharing the details of my intimate life, often with teens
and young adults, sometimes felt so vulnerable and wrong,

like I'd crossed a personal boundary. Being vulnerable to strangers and inevitably having portions of those talks end up in the press, sometimes misquoted, often left a pit in my stomach, as if I got caught naked in front of a crowd. I felt like I had betrayed the confidentiality of my family.

There's a Simpson's episode where Marge Simpson is teaching sex ed for a church youth group that Bart and his friends are attending. Bart is dying of humiliation and embarrassment while Marge tries to use finger puppets to encourage abstinence. Only after she brings Homer as a guest does the mere image of Homer and Marge touching each other gross out the teenagers so much that they rush to sign the "abstinence pledge" to get her to stop talking about their sex life.

That was my real life. Well, not the pledge part, but definitely the sex education in front of my own kids and their friends part. As a member of the speakers' bureau, I ended up, at one time or another, in every single one of my kids' high school classrooms talking about my life and sexually transmitted diseases. Every kid's nightmare.

All of this "sharing" through the speakers' bureau was taxing, exhausting really. But then I'd get letters. Through these years of baring my soul to students, I received many letters and notes from kids telling me their own stories of struggle and thanking me for giving them hope.

That's what kept me going. Those students are what made it worth doing at all.

My experience on the speakers' bureau prompted my greater involvement in AIDS advocacy and I began to attend and be a member of the Washington State Ryan White Care Act Advisory Board. After my trip to Washington, D.C., I was asked to participate and represent infected women on the board regarding state funding and legislation through Part 3 of the Act: *Women, Children, and Families infected and affected by HIV.*

These advisory group meetings were mediated by the Washington State Department of Health and took place every few months in South Seattle, not far from the airport. I was excited to learn about the issues being discussed and about legislation in the works that specifically applied to women and families.

I ended up participating on this board for several years, and our biggest victory was getting HIV testing for pregnant women in Washington State changed to opt-out instead of opt-in. What that meant was that HIV testing for a pregnant woman would not require a special form to be signed in order for the test to be performed, as it had been since the test was developed. Now, with the opt-out system, the HIV test became part of all mandatory tests for any pregnant woman. A person would have to sign a form *not* to receive it, effectively opting out.

When an HIV test is part of the battery of tests for pregnant women, a woman does not feel targeted or put in a position to disclose a particular risk when having to specifically ask to have the test performed.

With prenatal interventions and medications, the chance that HIV infection will be transmitted from an infected pregnant woman to her child can be reduced to 1 percent or less. But first, the woman and her doctor must know she is infected with HIV.

In reality, most infected women I met were like myself in that we had no idea we were HIV-positive or had been put at risk. Bottom line, most women didn't know that they should ask for this test.

Participating not only as a speaker but also as a member of this advisory/advocacy board solidified in my mind that there was still a very real need for quality HIV health education. That was what prompted me to go back to school. I'd been looking into a job at the health department, as a health educator. The job was everything I wanted to be doing; it was a shared position with Julie Z that included managing the speakers' bureau, presenting professional trainings about blood-borne pathogens, and focusing on the prevention of sexually transmitted infections in high-risk populations through partnerships with the department of corrections, drug rehab facilities, and youth shelters.

Before Christmas, while working my seasonal stint in retail, I began interviewing for the health department position. Interviewing for this job in the middle of holiday shopping, reminded me of why I wanted to work in healthcare even more. I hadn't had a job that required my college degree in over ten years. What made the job even more perfect for me was that, unlike the middle school teaching job, being HIV-positive in this position was an asset, not a liability. Who better to teach about sexually transmitted diseases, HIV, or blood-borne pathogens than a person who was managing those infections in real life? I found out I got the job in January.

When I took the job at the Health District, I wanted to be a provider, not a consumer, not a client, not a patient. Even before I went back to work, I would attend professional meetings about HIV, and people would come up to me thinking I was a pharmaceutical sales rep. I liked that. I dressed the part. I asked complicated medical questions. I wanted to be set apart in a different way other than being the woman with AIDS. It was a little messed up but that's how I felt. I was desperate to not have my identity completely tied to this disease.

In many ways, it was my privilege that allowed me to even play these roles, whether real or imaginary. The more "self-sufficient" I became, the more I created distance and disconnection from the community I was serving, the very community I'd needed desperately and been dependent on. I didn't process what was happening at the time, but, looking back, I think being set apart as an HIV provider only added to the broad hierarchy of privilege and power. I became part of one of the many systems that required "consumers" and, in a sense, depended on people being in need, but weren't always set up to give them power and independence. It's sad and embarrassing to see now how I wanted to be on top in that system. Because I could.

LIFE
WITH FOUR TEENAGERS

I am not young enough to know everything.

Oscar Wilde

Dale had been part of our family for two years when he and Teresa became high school seniors, Laura a sophomore, and Ryan an eighth grader. We had three teenage drivers, and our car insurance bill was larger than our food bill which was, in itself, humongous. The four of them snowboarded and we were fortunate to be able to get everyone season passes at Schweitzer Mountain. They had wakeboards and wetsuits; they had bikes, rollerblades, skateboards, summer camps, and football to keep them busy. And, apart from our time in Idaho at our cabin, we took family vacations during those years to Disneyland and Mexico. My kids were privileged kids. Our family was lucky. We tried to balance this life by instilling in our children that with privilege comes responsibility. I'm not sure we walked that line very well, but all of these teenagers had already seen a world of pain; the parent in me wanted to put some salve on that, to hope for some healing and let them simply enjoy life. I especially hoped that for Dale.

During those years, Scott was closer to Dale than I was. Dale's father had died when he was very young, and I think there was a big space to be the father figure in Dale's life. On the anniversary of Joyce's death, December 23, Scott, Dale, and the other kids would go skiing, which gave a lot of room for conversation and reflection while riding chairlifts. In the evening we would have Chris join us for dinner.

During their junior and senior year of high school, Teresa and Dale joined the speakers' bureau. They spoke as a team and would go to schools and other groups to give hour-long presentations about being affected by HIV and AIDS.

Between the two of them, they covered every means of transmission just by sharing their family stories. Dale's dad had been an IV drug user and was infected that way; Joyce was infected by having heterosexual sex; Kara was born infected; my brother Chris is gay; I had a blood transfusion. Pretty much covers it. They spoke quite often, were paid well, and became the most requested speakers on the bureau. Peer education—hearing from people who are the same age and whose lives look like yours—had been shown to be one of the most effective tools in HIV/AIDS prevention and education, and these two kids were nailing it.

A high school nurse once sent me a nice note about how effective Teresa and Dale were in their presentation. She said, "As I am sure you know, it is difficult to tell if teenagers are getting the message regarding AIDS and making healthy choices for their lives. As a nurse and an educator, I am frequently frustrated, feeling that I am not reaching my students. Dale and Teresa definitely reached them."

Laura and Ryan were not as verbal about our family dealing with HIV and didn't choose to be involved with the speakers' bureau. They did, however, at times use our AIDS story to make a point or to call someone out on being inappropriate. Unlike a lot of diseases, AIDS came with opinions, and teenagers often joked about behavior being "gay" and AIDS sometimes was a part of those demeaning slurs.

One night at a high school party, Laura heard a guy she didn't know putting down gay people and teasing someone that they were going to end up with AIDS. She looked at him dead face and in a serious monotone voice said, "My mom has AIDS."

"Are you fucking with me?" he asked back.

Right in his face, she straightforwardly replied, "I am not fucking with you."

Then her best friend backed her up: "She's totally not messing with you; her mom really does have AIDS."

Embarrassed and feeling like an idiot, he apologized profusely and hopefully learned something from the encounter.

Besides educating and defending HIV-positive people by bringing down the gavel and nailing someone, like Laura did at the party, my kids also found our AIDS story could be used in other ways. Sharing our story lent itself to deepening conversations and relationships but it also worked simply as an excuse to get out of something. I heard all my kids at one time or another on the phone telling someone, "No, I can't go tonight because my mom's not feeling good and I need to stay with her." This was occasionally true but often it was just an efficient way not to do something they didn't want to do.

Using our AIDS story for various personal reasons came to be known in our family as "pulling the AIDS card." We all pulled that card every now and then, even Scott.

I told all of them, including Dale, "This is something you can do. This is your life, your story. You can say whatever you want, whenever you want, about AIDS and our family. What you share is really your decision."

Then I would add, "But, my advice is that you save that card until it seems the most appropriate next step and not just as an excuse; it may be one of your very last options to explain yourself."

I'm pretty sure, in a backhanded kind of way, I'd just told my kids that they could use AIDS to help things go their way.

There were no guidebooks on how to be a good parent in the context of AIDS, teenagers, and dying from a feared disease. Scott and I were winging it for sure. I understood clearly that using our story for personal gain was a slippery slope that could lead to having a sort of victim mentality. I certainly didn't want that for my kids or for Dale.

But, this *was* our life and our story. Their story. And seriously, I didn't care if they did use it; they deserved at least that for all they were going through.

Apart from the overt ways the kids absorbed our HIV story into their middle- and high-school lives, overall, we had fun during those years. Family trips and events provided strong memories and relationships; investments in experiences at that time proved way more valuable than a new couch or updated kitchen. I had been a high school teacher and Scott worked with teens for many years, so we cherished this phase of parenting.

All of the kids found their own special activities and interests and it amazed me how each already was beginning to choose his or her own path. Ryan took his expertise in playing the guitar to a new level when he formed his first band in seventh grade. For the first time, he produced some original songs for his group and began brainstorming ways to promote his band's performances. They were excited when one of their youth leaders started a local "battle of the bands."

Laura, being a rescuer at heart, spent much time during

her teen years bringing home friends in need. She created her own "safe place," in our basement, a welcoming spot for friends to crash if they needed to. Almost every weekend, there was at least one stray teenager rolling out of bed for breakfast at our house. A few of her friends came to stay with us for extended periods during her high school years when they were going through tough times. Laura also loved animals and managed to talk us into several wayward cats and a cockatoo, who had to live in the bathroom half the time to avoid getting eaten by those cats.

Teresa and Dale often hung out with the same group of friends and were the most interested in school and sporting events of our bunch. They had fun planning a road trip to California with two of their close friends, making a detailed itinerary including staying with relatives along the way. At the end of the trip south, Scott met them on the Mexico border in California. We weren't quite comfortable with the idea of four kids going into a foreign country alone.

During that time of high school kids everywhere, I did have one rule. I'm not sure what I think about this now, but I told all the kids that they had to go to church. I told them, "I don't really care which church you go to, but you have to go somewhere." Because my faith in God was hugely helpful in dealing with my HIV, I hoped that my kids would find their version of that too.

We went to a church, Life Center, that all of them seemed to enjoy. The pastor had an easygoing, non-judgmental attitude and an amazing ability to talk to kids. We hijacked our own section in the balcony and often Laura and Teresa's friends would ask to come with us. At least half of those kids were nursing hangovers from the night before, but they would tag along anyway.

I'm not going to lie: we did bribe them! We promised that afterward we would go to Starbucks and order a crazy number of Frappuccinos. I miss that church; I have not been to one where I felt more at home since.

Our lives with four teenagers were definitely not perfect. Parenting is hard; parenting teenagers is really hard. I am not going to share all of the struggles my kids had during these years—those are their stories—but I will say they involved alcohol, drugs, boyfriends and girlfriends, arguments, running away and coming back, yelling, cussing, crying, and a whole lot of talking things out.

It's hard growing up. It's harder growing up in a blended family of any kind. Trying to find your place and be who you want to be, an individual who is evolving, while also fitting into the whole of your family is a difficult task. Whether you are the parent or the child, I guess the goal is to make it out of adolescence alive and still loving each other. We chose to laugh and survive the drama together. I would call that a success.

INDEPENDENCE DAY

Promise you'll remember:
You're braver than you believe
and stronger than you seem,
and smarter than you think.

A.A. Milne

The summer of 2002 started with Teresa and Dale graduating from high school. It was a very exciting time, not only for our family but for the whole neighborhood because ours were the oldest kids on the block, and this was the first graduation. My neighbor, Di, put on a very nice graduation party, and the whole neighborhood came with thoughtful gifts. Both Teresa and Dale were set to start college at the University of Washington in the fall, so several of the gifts had UW themes.

On the night of graduation, we all went to Dale's Grandma's house to take photos with his family. Looking at those photos now, there are quite a variety of people in them; they are a snapshot of what our life was like at the time. There was our family, Dale, his grandma, and his brother Chris—all of that makes sense. But then in almost all of the pictures is a friend who had been living in our basement for several weeks after some trauma in her own family. Those photos remind me that, at the time, we had a fluid home; people came and went. Some people might think this was a little nuts, especially given my health challenges, but for us, it was an easy choice. We kept an open door for those in need, and we don't regret it.

After graduation, the kids got summer jobs and we, as usual, began to spend a lot of time at the cabin. Teresa and Dale's friends came up to the lake on several occasions, enjoying hikes and spending lazy days out in the boat. They were relishing the last days of high school, feeling that era closing as they split toward their different colleges and universities.

I started to notice Dale was distancing himself from us. One day I heard him talking on the phone, chatting about our family like we were mere acquaintances. When I asked him about this later, he didn't say much. I had read that kids do this kind of distancing when they are ready to go off on their own. They crave independence; it all seemed pretty normal. Then, one random day in July, I was hanging out at home when Dale came into my bedroom and said, "I have decided to move out."

Confused, I asked him, "Oh really, when?"

"Today, in an hour. A truck is coming to get my stuff."

An hour later a truck pulled up and he moved all his personal belongings to a friend's house. I was shocked. I had thought of Dale as a member of our family and I didn't see this coming.

Joyce had promised Dale independence, that he could be on his own when he turned eighteen, and he was taking her up on that promise and spreading his wings. Even though Dale hadn't told us in advance, I'd seen it coming. He was restless. But I wasn't ready for such an abrupt departure. It took some time to process that we were, indeed, back to our original family of five.

Dale started college at the University of Washington in the fall. I still saw him when he spoke for the speakers' bureau since I remained the director of the bureau through my position at the health department. We got along fine during those times and sometimes even joked about how, for a couple of years, I was his substitute mom.

The truth was, we were all broken to one degree or another; I don't think there was enough glue, not enough well-meaning goodwill, to put the pieces back together.

DAD

Sometimes only one person is missing,
and the whole world seems depopulated.

Alphonse de Lamartine

In the fall of 2002, when Teresa started college, Scott was traveling a lot, having taken a new job with an organization focused on international development. One weekend in September, when everyone else was out of town, my dad, who had been fishing in Montana, stopped in Spokane to stay overnight before heading home. I had Dad all to myself, which hadn't happened in a very long time. We went to church together and then I talked him into going to a matinee, My Big Fat Greek Wedding. Mom never really liked going to the movie theater, especially when they began to get expensive, so this was a big treat for him, really for both of us.

Dad had his fiftieth college anniversary in October. He'd been on the committee that planned the celebration for their class from Eastern State College, now called Eastern Washington University, and was super excited about the festivities. The weekend overflowed with fun events including a football game at the university and a big fancy dinner and dance at the nicest hotel in Spokane, the newly restored Davenport.

On Sunday, when all of their activities were over, he and Mom decided they would stay at our house before traveling back to their home on the west side of the state. Scott had left on a work trip to California, so I was happy to have the company. That afternoon Dad took Ryan, Laura, and me out to Red Robin for lunch. Mom frowned and pouted a bit when he defiantly ordered the tower of onion rings and devoured them with my kids. She'd worked so hard to keep him on his diabetic diet, but he was in no mood to comply, even laughing a little in her face while he was licking his lips.

That night, Sunday night, we were watching TV and I was actually snuggling with Dad on the couch when he brought up Dale. I was feeling like a bit of a failure because our guardianship had ended so abruptly.

Dad said a couple of encouraging things about how our hearts were in a good place when we brought Dale into our home and reminded me of all the fun times we'd had with him that would live on, regardless. Lastly, he said, "Just focus on your own kids now."

I had a lot of peace after that conversation. I had no idea that it would be the last time we would ever have a meaningful talk.

The next morning my parents were supposed to drive home. Dad woke up, drank two cups of coffee, said goodbye to Laura and Ryan as they headed off to school, and then went downstairs to get dressed. I went upstairs to get ready for work.

A few minutes later, Mom was at the door of my bathroom. She looked at me casually and said, "I think your dad is having a stroke."

I tried to take in what she was saying as her face didn't match the seriousness of the statement. "I'll call 911," I said back.

"I don't think we need an ambulance," replied Mom, still seeming disconnected.

"I'll let them decide that." I dialed the number into my phone.

Dad was taken by ambulance to Deaconess Medical Center. He'd lost the ability to form intelligible words but the whole time in the ER he tried to keep talking, being especially irritated that he couldn't remove his wedding ring or his prized blue star-sapphire ring on the other hand because both were swelling. It distracted me and gave me hope he would be okay.

I knew several of the medical staff and doctors in the emergency room, having been there myself or with my friends on several occasions. It felt good to recognize faces, but by far the one I was the most relieved to see was Dr. C. He'd heard from someone we were there, dropped everything, and come to evaluate Dad's MRI results.

One of the things I've always liked about Dr. C is his frankness and honesty. Even when it's terrible news, at least I have a chance to prepare. But that day I wasn't at all prepared for his diagnosis.

With a very grim demeanor, he said, "Your dad is going to die. It might not be today, but it will be soon. The bleed in his brain is too big; it can't be fixed. I'm so sorry."

Dad lost consciousness in the elevator going to ICU. His last two words miraculously came out clearly. He looked at Mom and said, "I'm sorry."

I'll never forget that. I can hear it in my mind still and can see the very sad look he had in his eyes as he shut them for the final time and slipped into a coma.

My brothers and sister drove as fast as they could from Seattle and made it to his hospital room at around four that afternoon. Dad died thirty minutes later; he was seventy-two years old.

That was one of the saddest days of my life. Our family

has never fully recovered from his death. Dad was our center, and without him, we spun out into our own private lives.

There are so many things I could say about that day: how I think he could hear everything we said even though he was unconscious; how Debbie, again, was with me all day helping me care for Mom who was definitely in shock; how Pat and Debbie sprung into action making our family and friends a spaghetti dinner that night; how we can endure much more than we can imagine when all of a sudden we are the one in charge of a trauma, pulling it together to call everyone involved and helping them to make a plan.

Mom did not go home. We drove right to Wenatchee, our family town and the place Dad had been superintendent of schools for seventeen years. We buried him there on a hill overlooking the high school he had helped build. He died on Monday, and his memorial was five days later on Saturday. Hundreds of people came, most of them teachers and staff who'd worked with him over the years. He was buried in the very clothes he'd left home with, the clothes that were in his suitcase.

After the funeral, my sister and I took Mom home. It was so weird to walk into their house and see Dad's stuff everywhere: his glasses on the table, his books and jewelry on his nightstand, his forms filled out for a men's church retreat. He'd gone intending to return; everything was exactly where he had left it. Looking at it all, things that surrounded my dad's life, his stuff, reminded me of him, smelled like him. All his things were in waiting, as if expecting him to return and continue using them. It broke my heart.

When my sister and I left to go back home, a week later, we left Mom alone in that house. That moment began a turning point. I felt like I was now the parent abandoning my child to conquer the world on her own. From that day on

I felt responsible for her. She would go on to live seventeen more years, by herself.

Death is hard. By this point in my life, I had dealt with and experienced death quite often. But sudden death, death without warning, death with no goodbyes, no resolutions, no preparation—that kind of death is horrible. I woke up one morning thinking it would be a typical day, but then, that day became etched in my head, every detail burned into my memory for the rest of my life. That kind of loss requires so much mental and emotional grieving after the fact. After Dad died, I was shaken to the core. I was tired. I lost about ten pounds from not eating. I was sad. So, so sad.

I often think back to that last conversation we had. It was a pure gift to me, a turning point of sorts, a definitive moment in my life when I just started moving forward, intentionally, focusing on my future and no longer dwelling on the past.

After Dale moved out and Dad died, a weird little thing happened that has stuck with Teresa and me for years. We'd put a hummingbird feeder outside the kitchen window, above the sink. For years, we never saw a hummingbird, but then they started coming. I noticed them and so did Teresa. We were deep in confusion and grief at the time; confronted with how, emotionally, to deal with more loss, it was hard to know how to process it all.

Then the hummingbirds. One day we decided that maybe the hummingbirds came to give us hope. Hope for our future, hope for our family, and hope for my mom who now lived alone. In the many years since, Teresa and I have given each other many hummingbird-themed gifts, reminding us that there is always hope, but also, that we are resilient, and we are survivors.

They also remind us that we are family and will always be there for each other, no matter what happens.

And ... God ... how I miss my dad.

SEATTLE

Every new beginning comes
from some other beginning's end.

Lucius Annaeus Seneca

W hen Scott returned to working in youth ministries and management in the summer of 2003, we talked about our desire to get back to the west side of Washington State where many of our family lived, where Teresa was now at school at the University of Washington, and where the kids would have more opportunities as they pursued college and jobs. To be honest, I was ready to leave Spokane. I was ready to start fresh, and move past being the AIDS lady who taught in schools.

It was almost Thanksgiving so I reasoned that the best plan would be for Scott to go back and forth to the Seattle area with his new job while Laura, Ryan, and I stayed in Spokane so they could both finish the school year. I figured we could all move in the upcoming summer after Laura graduated.

That was the plan. Yet, one day in late October, I started wondering how our house would fare in the real estate market so I got out a flimsy little "For Sale" sign from our garage and placed it next to our driveway in front of our house.

I was working a split shift at the health department that day, so I went home to make dinner between working at my office and my shift at the shelter downtown. In the middle of boiling noodles, my cell phone rang.

"Hello," I said.

"Hi. I'm wondering how much you are asking for your house?" said a woman.

"Ummmmm. One hundred and seventy-five thousand, I think," I replied, hoping that was right.

"Well, I'd love to come and see it," she said.

"When?" I asked.

"I'm sitting in your driveway; can I come through right now?"

I looked around the house. I had two teenagers in full control of the house that day. I'd not been home since early morning. The house was more than disheveled. I stared at dishes, the ingredients for a spaghetti dinner, backpacks, and books strewn everywhere around the kitchen.

Oh, whatever ... I had put the sign out hours earlier as a test; might as well see what this woman would think.

"Sure," I replied, "but I have been gone all day, and it's a mess. I need to go back to work in ten minutes, so I won't be able to walk you through. But if you want to look around yourself, come on in."

A beautiful young woman appeared at my door, and I gave her full range of my very lived-in house.

Five minutes later she came back into my kitchen and said, "I want to buy your house."

Later I asked her what it was that attracted her to my dirty house. She said, "I have three boys. I walked in and the house seemed full of warmth and smelled like spaghetti. I thought that I could see us living here."

So much for staging, homemade cookies, and perfection ... if you want to sell your house, throw out some laundry and textbooks and make spaghetti!

We were moving, and we were moving quickly. I would see people even a year later from Spokane who would say, "You moved?" We did not have farewell parties, we did not send out Christmas cards, and we did not leave with any fanfare. We just packed up everything we had collected after thirteen years in Spokane and moved.

SACRED
CIRCUMSTANCES AND
TRIVIAL COINCIDENCES

Coincidence is God's way of remaining anonymous.

Albert Einstein

'm a believer in what I call sacred circumstances. This refers to the many choices—big and small—that, had they been different, would have profoundly changed the direction of my life.

I first started thinking about this around fifteen years ago when I was studying the book of Esther, in the Old Testament. Esther is a particularly interesting book; it's the only book in the Bible that never mentions God even though it's all about the plight of the Jewish people and their captivity. I've owned the same Bible for almost twenty years, and I often write or underline in it. When I was studying Esther, I made some underlines in the footnotes.

The footnotes say, "This verse marks the literary center of the narrative. When things could not look worse, a series of seemingly trivial coincidences marks a critical turn that brings resolution to the story."

And then later on in the notes: "Circumstances that seemed incidental earlier in the narrative take on crucial significance." (NIV Study Bible.)

Our "sacred circumstances" kicked off when our house sold in a matter of hours in late October 2003, and then the same week, I got a call from the Seattle School District informing me that if Ryan showed up to classes on December 8, he could have a spot at the school he wanted, Roosevelt High School. Ryan had been at the bottom of their waitlist, but she called the long line of people above us and nobody wanted to move in December. This meant we had a very short amount of time between Ryan's first day at Roosevelt and finding a Seattle house to live in.

Moving from Spokane to Seattle in December of 2003 put us in an impossible housing market. The average price per square foot of houses in Seattle was about triple what it was in the Spokane market. We quickly realized that we were going to have to downsize dramatically to move into the city.

The criteria for our house hunt included one crucial requirement: we needed a cement basement where Ryan could make music as loud as he wanted without the neighbors calling the police for unwanted noise as we had experienced on numerous occasions in Spokane when his band sometimes practiced in our garage.

We began to look at houses to buy, which brought us to a house on a dead end that was for sale. Coincidentally, a rental house was having an open house next door, so we decided to check it out. Scott didn't make it past the living room; he just stopped and ended up in a conversation with the owner, a lovely woman named Sharon. They mostly talked about the organization Scott worked for since her son had just returned from one of their camps.

That house was so small, I didn't think twice about it until Sharon called us in Spokane. The first question I asked was, "How did you get our phone number?"

She said that Scott's office had given it to her. Sharon was calling to say that she thought she was supposed to rent her house to us. She said, "I've never had such a distinct feeling; I just can't stop thinking that I'm supposed to rent my house to you."

I replied, "That's kind of you, but we actually can't afford your rent and we really want to buy a house."

Sharon continued, "I thought that might be the case. I'd like to offer it to you on a month-to-month contract so you can continue to look for a house to buy. Oh, and I want to reduce the rent by four hundred dollars a month to make it more affordable."

Then she added, "You know, I'm not a particularly religious person but I just feel like God is telling me to rent my house to you."

We rented Sharon's house.

Other things lined up in record time. Laura was a senior but was in a college "running start" program where her college class credits transferred to her Spokane high school. We found out that all of the Washington State community colleges would transfer her credits, so for winter and spring quarters she would attend North Seattle Community College and still be able to graduate with her friends in Spokane at the end of the school year.

I began to feel a sense of peace in the midst of the chaos of moving. Not just moving, but moving fast, in the middle of the school year, with teenagers, at Christmastime. It felt like God was orchestrating the small details. It felt like we were in step with a bigger plan.

December 16, 2003, was my last day in Spokane. Dale was a speaker at Lewis and Clark High School and, as the director of the speakers' bureau, I was with him all day. Laura and I had stayed in town after Scott and Ryan moved a week earlier to Seattle because we needed to finish school and work.

I came to work with my car packed, so after finishing with Dale's presentations at the high school, Laura said goodbye to her best friend, Gabe, and we got in the car and left for Seattle. As I watched Dale walk away that day, it was such a visual declaration that a chapter was ending.

Laura and I made our way over Snoqualmie Pass in the dark, navigating the worst snowstorm I'd ever driven in; it was treacherous. We finally arrived in Seattle and found our neighborhood. As we rounded the corner of our new street a flurry of colorful Christmas lights welcomed us, shining all the way up the road on almost every house.

It felt like we were home.

END OF AN ERA

There is sacredness in tears.
They are not the mark of weakness, but of power. They
speak more eloquently than ten thousand tongues.
They are the messengers of overwhelming grief,
of deep contrition, and of unspeakable love.

Washington Irving

After being a part of it for more than nine years, the Spokane HIV/AIDS Speakers' Bureau had become a family to me. A family that experienced trauma, grief, and loss. Years later, meeting with people who survived it, even my friend Julie Z, who led the group but was not infected, reminded me that this was a unique and special time in our lives and carried with it a mountain of intense feelings and memories. It was an era when we were thrown together in a battle and somehow a few of us were lucky enough to survive. But the losses were many; the body count was high.

I understand why people who face mortal danger together form a bond that lasts a lifetime. Our 1990s HIV community in Spokane has that bond. It was truly a battle we fought together and many were lost along the way. It's been years since the height of the AIDS epidemic and yet, when we get together, it feels like it was yesterday. When we see each other now, there are things that just don't need to be said.

That season of our lives will never fade because to let it fade would be to let them fade, to forget.

We will never forget the loss.

PART 3

TOO OLD TO DIE YOUNG

GAP YEAR

To everything, there is a season,
and a time to every purpose under heaven.

Ecclesiastes 3:1 NKJV

My garden has taught me the importance of seasons. There are the obvious seasons: winter, spring, summer, fall ... but then there are also seasons of life. There are seasons when you have energy to do all that work in your yard, seasons to hire someone, seasons to plant a vegetable garden, and then there are seasons to just throw out some wildflower seeds. The point of seasons is to learn to be flexible, to learn not to beat yourself up, to learn to let things go and sometimes to try things that are new.

...I needed a break—a break from my own life. I needed a season with no concrete plans, no clear path, just space. I needed to catch my breath, to clear my mind. I felt like I was suffocating; I needed to come up for air.

I related to the high school senior who is just not quite ready to start college. I wanted to be the kid who graduates and then takes the next year off. They call it a "gap year." I desperately needed a gap year.

I took that gap year, and then another, and another. That "gap" went on in some capacity for years. I didn't talk about HIV publicly or give a speech about AIDS for ten years, not until April 2014.

My "break" from health education and advocacy was almost a break-up.

When we settled in Seattle, after getting through that first Christmas, I felt lost with no job and very few people in my life. I had only a few friends in Seattle. Most lived in areas that required at least a half-hour drive.

In January, I joined a women's Bible study. As I tried to describe my life and what I did in Spokane to these new acquaintances, none of the women seemed to relate to what I was sharing. I would be lying to say that I didn't try to make myself sound important, telling them about all of the large groups I had given speeches to on the speakers' bureau. That they were not impressed would be an understatement. It was humbling but also what I had wanted, right? To be a normal person? Not special?

Well, I got what I wished for.

The one place I landed was at the University of Washington as a mentor for a college Bible study group. For some reason, this was where I felt most comfortable even though I was well into my forties, and they were twenty-year-olds. It seemed like every week we were all trying to answer the question, "What am I supposed to do with my life?"

I didn't have too many answers for these students, but I enjoyed being in the middle of the process with each one. I ended up being a mentor off and on for almost ten years, and many of my mentees are now deep into their thirties and have become friends.

Our whole family was in transition through those first years in Seattle; most of those life changes proved to be adventurous and fun. My kids were growing up, finding their own lives, and defining who they wanted to be as individuals. In a way, I was doing the same thing.

I wondered, "Apart from HIV, who am I?"

Scott worked for three different nonprofit organizations during my gap years. One centered on human rights and abuses, one on land rights. Both of those were about laws and litigation to help change the plight of people in under-resourced communities, especially women and children. The third organization also had some focus internationally, helping to develop community partnerships. He ended up traveling the globe with these positions, meeting a variety of interesting people and learning about their cultures and customs. He also found himself witnessing poverty on a level he could not have imagined.

Our whole family was learning about the world, not just Scott. All of the kids lived abroad during these years with school and jobs. Between the three of them, they spent significant time in India, Ireland, Italy, South Africa, Japan, and Mexico. I was lucky to be able to hop on a plane and join a few of their adventures.

One of Scott's jobs landed us in Washington, D.C., for three and a half years. Compared to the Northwest, everything felt formal. We found ourselves wearing suits quite often. The dress code at Scott's new job was "business formal." We didn't even know the rules of dressing before we moved to D.C. In Seattle, "business casual" is about as formal as it gets!

Not long after we arrived, I planned to go to a Sunday matinee with one of Scott's co-workers. She called me right before I left the house and said, "Oh, I just wanted you to know that I'm wearing jeans."

I'm thinking, "Ya. Duh. What else would you wear to a movie?"

Out loud I said, "You know, I'm from Seattle. You never have to tell us when to wear jeans." Then with a chuckle, I added, "You only have to tell us when to dress up."

This woman and a few others that worked in Scott's office invited me to be in a women's support group. It wasn't exactly a Bible study, although we talked about the Bible and a few other books. It was genuinely a group to encourage women. They called themselves the Gorillas, and I loved these women.

The name Gorillas originated on a work retreat, which, as Scott's spouse, I was graciously invited to. That weekend I learned more about the organization's work and strategy, tackling injustices including bonded slavery and other human rights violations around the world. The day ended with hot tubbing, some wine drinking, and a long walk in the foggy woods.

On that cloudy walk, one of us said, "It's like we're gorillas in the mist!" The title from the movie about Dian Fossey's life became our inspiration, and we were promptly named the Gorillas!

The organization they worked for was faith-based, and every workday at eleven, they participated in a corporate prayer time for half an hour at the office. These women had a variety of opinions about "eleven o'clock prayer" but my favorite discussions centered around what the twenty-something interns asked the group to pray for.

One of the Gorillas snarkily asked, "Does God really care about parking spaces?"

And we laughed.

One of their jobs was to set up safe houses for kids, as young as five years old, who had been trafficked. It didn't feel like any of our problems were big enough to be "God-worthy" in light of the terrible human rights abuses that were daily addressed by this organization.

That group of incredibly smart, savvy Gorillas was the highlight of my years in D.C. Watching them navigate their faith while not giving in to the patriarchy and the Christian cliches taught me to be bold and to stand up for the female version of God. They reminded me often that God is just as much female as male. The female side of God was often ignored or overlooked.

We could just as easily and truly be praying to Mother God as Father God. Their ideas of faith broadened my own, and their clever wittiness taught me to laugh, even when things seemed hard or unfair.

And the wine ... that was great too.

MAGIC JOHNSON

Never, never, never give up.

Winston Churchill

I wrote a letter to Magic Johnson right after he was diagnosed as HIV-positive. I don't remember exactly what I said but it was mostly a thank-you card of sorts, telling him that his courage to speak publicly was inspirational and that his positive viewpoint had led me to the gym, to new personal goals.

He didn't respond—I mean why would he? What would he have said: "Congratulations on going to the gym twice a week!"?

One of my favorite memories when we were living in Washington, D.C., was the day Teresa and I met Magic Johnson! We were at an event for World AIDS Day, and we heard that he was going to be speaking. We happened to be in a seminar put on by the ONE Campaign earlier in the day, and we met someone who heard our story and said that they could get us in the front of the line to meet Magic. This was before cell phones had cameras, so we immediately ran out to the CVS and bought a disposable camera. Then we went to listen to Magic Johnson's presentation.

Magic talked about his kids and said that at one point, early on, after his diagnosis, he was afraid that he wouldn't see them grow up. This deeply resonated with me. I experienced so much sadness and grief when I thought about my future in those early days. I wanted to stay in the moment and be appreciative when the kids were young after my initial diagnosis, but it was hard not to peer into the future and focus on what I would miss when I died, all the special moments and occasions where I wouldn't be present.

Afterward, we made our way to the VIP meet and greet area and, as promised, were first in line. I don't think I was prepared for the man, Magic Johnson, to be standing next to me. He was grander in stature than my imagination had accounted for but even more monumental in personality with his kind eyes and smile.

After we were introduced, I gave him a hug and said, "I related so much to what you were talking about. I had fears about not seeing my kids grow up too, but now I'm planning my daughters' weddings! I never imagined I would live to do that. Even crazier is the fact that I fully expect to help raise my grandkids one day."

He smiled and said, "That's so great," in his gracious tone, then Teresa and I got a photo and one of my bucket list items was checked.

That short interaction with Magic reminded me that I was in unknown territory. I had hoped and prayed to see my kids grow up, and here I was looking at kids in their twenties. I hadn't put a lot of thought into this phase of life because I never imagined making it this far, living this long. As it turned out, my favorite part of my quiet years after we moved to Seattle and D.C. was the time I had with my kids. During those years they became adults, and when they weren't exploring other parts of the world, Scott and I would spend as much time as possible with each of them. There were college graduations, marriages, lots of travel, and new careers. These were the pre-baby days that included many late nights. I loved going out to bars and pubs with my now legal-aged children and their significant others, listening to them plan their lives. I even enjoyed it when they would tell Scott and me how they were going to do everything better than we did.

I would think, "More power to you, kid!" Truth is, I agreed with almost all of their assessments of our flaws. Since having their own kids, all three have been much more gracious and forgiving about their parents' shortcomings.

At one time or another, each of our kids landed back at our house for temporary housing during different transitions. As much as I adore my grandkids, the time we had with our grown children and their significant others in those years, before they had kids and mortgages, was priceless.

All three of them eventually became parents. I am now the grandma to six beautiful children, the biggest miracle and the farthest-off dream I'd been willing to allow myself. Having reached that pinnacle, I'm now having to rewrite my hopes for the future to include the grandkids' life moments, their graduations, careers, and weddings! I had never dared to hope, let alone imagine, that I might be present for any of these moments.

I go back in my mind to a conversation with Scott, right after I was diagnosed. We were having a difficult conversation about moving on after I died. I told him there was no way I wanted him and the kids to be alone after I died. I wanted him to feel free to fall in love and marry someone else.

I did add, "I mean, you could wait a little while after I die."

I also asked him if he could please have a prenup so that all of the money from our lawsuit settlement would be allocated to our kids and not his potential new spouse's family.

Looking back on that time, preparing for his future, it's weird to think that if I had died within that three-to-five-year period, Scott could now potentially have been remarried to someone else for the last twenty-five years. My six grandkids might be calling some other woman grandma right now.

I think that's what Magic was getting to that day as he spoke. You can talk about wanting to see your kids grow up in a speech and hope the audience is understanding. But unless you yourself have lived believing that time with your children has a rapidly approaching expiration date, you really don't know the gravity and depth of that longing.

Of all my life achievements and goals, the thing I am happiest about was something I had no control over. I lived. I was given days and years to see my family grow—and for that, I'm extremely grateful.

DEPRESSION
AND COPING

Life is a battle;
may we all be enabled to fight it well.

Charlotte Brontë

I thought we were fine. We looked good from the outside, but then as we settled into a new space in a new city, as we let our guard down from the constant exposure of public speaking and Christian leadership roles, the truth started to surface and expose cracks in our mental health. Like sunlight exposing a layer of dust on my glass lamps—a dull patina sits where I thought they would glimmer.

This would describe my life and my marriage around our twenty-fifth anniversary. Life was stabilizing on the health front; the kids were now adults; the baby of the family was in college. It was maybe the first moment in a very long time, in years of being together, that it was just Scott and me. The two of us. Not only the two of us, but the two of us with no major problems or issues. Imagining ourselves to be "fine," we ran smack dab into midlife and were forced to look at all of the unimaginable shit that we'd been stuffing for many years.

Managing illness over a long time is overwhelming, and to keep up with kids, jobs, and appearances, we did what we could to get by. What we didn't notice or realize were the issues we were not dealing with when we were in survival mode. I think this can happen with any major issue that forces a family to cope in this way, not just chronic disease management and loss.

In survival mode, I failed to see what was wrong because our "coping" life became our normal life. I stopped noticing how Scott and I were responding to each other as a couple, how we were handling the stress and responsibility of additional "family" members, how we were processing losing friends and loved ones, and who we were choosing to process all of this with when it wasn't each other.

We found ourselves in marriage counseling. I thought a lot about my journey up to that point and saw clearly that a theme of my pilgrimage had been and continued to be depression.

For me, depression feels tired. I don't feel strong; I don't feel connected or able to focus very well. I feel like a ship that is out of fuel and drifting at sea. Did I mention I feel tired? Overwhelmingly tired. I am exhausted even when I'm doing nothing. I get scared that this is forever who I am, that I'm stuck. I feel like a rabbit hole is sucking me down, like I need help but often reject the help that's offered. I am alone. I don't like being alone but find it hard to engage with anyone, even if they are right next to me.

I've struggled with it off and on my whole life. Some years, some phases of life, are just harder than others.

Once, I read about a counselor who tells all her patients dealing with depression to try to do four things every day: get up, make your bed, shower, and get dressed. Those were habits I started every day when we were in marriage counseling. I mean, I understood the concept—the idea that getting ready for your day makes it less likely to go back to bed, less likely to never get up, and less likely to never leave the house. Some days this has helped me, but then, I'm not beyond taking a nap, or going back to bed in my clothes.

Through dealing with depression and really all things that have been out of control in my life, I've learned how important my faith is to me, how important God is to me. I thought about how I wanted to stop performing for God, stop trying to "earn" love, and to just be a person who is loved. I didn't come to God to be right or even to be just. I came to God because I needed to be loved. I needed to learn how to love. And maybe that had to start with me learning how to love myself. Learning to have love for myself and see myself as the person whom God felt was worthy to be loved. Only from there could I see how everyone else just needed to be loved, too.

Most of us in the Lewis family have undergone some kind of therapy. I've become a big fan of counseling; I like to think of it as similar to getting a tune-up up on your car. Regular maintenance prevents having to do a major overhaul, whether it's the vehicle I drive or the vehicle of my soul.

One time, after hearing the story of growing up with AIDS in our family, one of my kid's counselors paused and then said, "That's a whole lot of coping."

I have never, in one sentence, heard our life story summed up so well. It was, and continues to be, a whole lot of coping. Coping that over time came out sideways in many forms: depression, anxiety, addiction, perfectionism, bitterness, sadness, and control. The list is long and varied. It didn't always come out badly. I think some of our best ideas and efforts as a family have also come from this coping. A fictional book I read recently about the AIDS epidemic and the people who survived insinuated that the best an HIV-positive person could expect or hope for was "good scarring."

The good scars. We want scars that show character, not ones that are hard for people to look at.

I wish I had a dollar for every time I've said to myself, "You're going to be okay."

This is my self-talk when I'm trying to calm down. Believe me, thirty years of managing this disease has required a tremendous amount of coping and self-talk. I have a lot of fears about medicine and health issues. Everything from allergies requiring Benadryl, to choking on things, to numbness in my hands and feet, dizziness or vertigo, to not remembering things. My go-to calming mechanism is my internal voice saying, "You're going to be okay." Sometimes it works better than others.

I also tell myself to "breathe in, breathe out," managing anxiety around just getting through my day. Most people have no idea that this is happening because I am so good, so practiced, at making everything appear to be fine.

I'm not even sure what bad scarring looks like when it's internal. I do know it's different for each person, and it is hard to hide. The same book about HIV, when talking about a long-term AIDS survivor, called him the world's luckiest man while being the unluckiest too.

Surviving ... Was it a blessing? For sure. And a burden? Absolutely. Neither will cease to be true until the day I die.

Teresa said something that I believe, after years of coping, seems to ring true. She said, "When I was a kid I felt pretty messed up and I get, like, it was unusual. The older I get, the more I see that it isn't special to be messed up. It seems like everybody has problems."

The truth is, we are all minor tragedies, and we all must learn to cope.

I've found that one of the best ways to move forward is to start where I am and with what I have. Waiting for things to line up, waiting for a better day, or waiting for a better situation—well, that day may never come. So today I choose to get out of bed and start anew with what I have and try to make something good come from it. Maybe something will happen and maybe it won't, but I'm going to choose to love myself and others regardless.

That's how we defy the prognosis and beat the odds.

BOTTLES OF PILLS

Medicine is not only a science; it is also an art.
It does not consist of compounding pills and plasters;
it deals with the very processes of life,
which must be understood before they may be guided.

Paracelsus

Once I was prescribed an HIV medication with side effects similar to psychedelic drugs. The doctor told me to take the pills before I went to bed and warned me that I would be having some wild, vivid dreams. He was right. I never slept well when I was on that drug.

Back when I was working in retail, I spaced out and took this drug right before I went to work. First of all, there is no way I should have driven anywhere that day; thankfully I made it safely to a parking lot downtown before it kicked in. Secondly, going to a sales job while your mind is in an altered state is never a good idea. But I needed that job, and I was there before I realized what I'd done. It was a long, intense day. I remember being uncertain which customers I had already talked to, how to operate the till with so many codes, and wondering if the words coming out of my mouth were making sense. I was lucky to be working with a woman who covered for me most of my shift.

I have a relationship with my medicine. It's difficult to describe a relationship with an inanimate object, but I've come to realize it's something that people who deal with chronic illness or cancer often understand. I brought this up with my sister-in-law who is battling leukemia and taking a shitload of medicine right now. She hates her medicine but is well aware that taking it regularly is one of her only hopes to beat this cancer. I laughed about having relationships with medicine, and she chuckled, relieved to realize that she wasn't alone in feeling the love/hate towards her pills.

I want to establish strongly that it's a complete privilege to have access to the medications that have kept me alive. There are many places around the world where HIV-positive people would give anything for the options and variety of pharmaceutical drugs that I have had available and accessible in treating my HIV infection. This whole chapter is a story that many people would love to be telling you.

Nonetheless, managing multiple medications and their side effects can be extremely challenging.

After I began taking AZT, I noticed that I was thinking and feeling things towards my medicine, like you would think and feel towards an actual person. It was a love-hate relationship. I loved that my medicine kept me alive; that was the goal after all. But I absolutely hated the pit in my stomach every day when I looked at those bottles of pills and thought about taking them. Even anticipating taking them made me anxious. I dreaded the side effects sure to accompany those pills being in my body, nausea and fatigue being the worst.

Many days I'd stare at my bottles of prescription drugs for so long that I'd come back later and wonder, had I taken the meds, or had I just thought about taking them?

That's when I got a pill dispenser with sections and compartments for different days and times. It was a good way to keep track of whether I had taken my meds or not. I definitely needed that. I think those little contraptions were developed and marketed for old people who forget things, but my relationship with medicine started when I was thirty-two years old and newly diagnosed.

Managing medicine requires not only the mind but also the participation of one's emotional and psychological self. Handling the side effects of a drug by adding another drug often creates more issues and more side effects. It's a vicious cycle, one medication leading to another. Over time, with experience, I've successfully limited these extra medications, but as I get older and am dealing with typical aging issues, like high blood pressure and elevated cholesterol, I'm having to compromise and consider adding more medication to my daily routine.

Since 1990, I've taken over sixty thousand pills to stay alive. It is the greatest blessing and the greatest challenge. Medicine has put a stress on my body for years but has also kept me alive.

COLLATERAL DAMAGE

*Collateral Damage is described as
unintentional or accidental damage
to people or things that happen
as a result of an action or event;
they are damages that were not meant to happen.*

Janis Waldman

As I think of those early days of AIDS, I am reminded that all of the children, infected and affected, are the collateral damage. They have the saddest stories, and they are the saddest part of the story.

Recently, on the AIDS Memorial Instagram page, I read a story about two women who grew up with parents who died of AIDS. Their dad was infected by a blood transfusion and by the time he was diagnosed, their mom was also HIV-positive. Their parents decided not to tell anyone, wanting to avoid the stigma and possible job loss from disclosing their HIV status.

In telling the story, their daughter talked about how hard it was for her and her sister to keep a family secret with the AIDS tragedy unfolding every day around them. She did her best for years until her mind and body rebelled and began to make her physically sick.

I felt for her parents, having had to make these hard decisions about disclosure for our own children. On one hand, as a parent, trying to protect your family from stigma and, on the other, giving your child an outlet to process HIV in a bigger community. There wasn't always an obvious best choice.

This was just one story from the kids who lived and died through the AIDS epidemic in the early days. Kids who kept their families' HIV secrets, who were discriminated against whether they were infected or not. Kids who inherited complicated adult problems and issues, plopped into their laps at incredibly young ages. Kids who grew up way too fast, having to be the caregivers. Kids, like Chris and Dale, who suffered great loss, not only in losing family members, but also having to resettle and rebuild their lives in other places, as children.

Some of these kids have had difficult adult lives with addictions of all types. Some were so young when their moms and dads died that they don't remember them. Some have relatives who rarely discuss the family member who died of AIDS because they're still afraid of the stigma. Kids grew up alone and lonely. Some were split up from their siblings and placed in foster care. One of these kids I know, whose mom died, is now an adult and has become HIV-positive himself.

My own kids did not come out of this unscathed. Every single one of my now-adult children has some level of anxiety. My kids stuffed a lot of feelings they did not have the tools to process and they all worried. Experiences like these in childhood have effects that last for years and express themselves in multiple ways. From a very early age, my kids learned that terrible things can happen. So I understand now why they worry about other terrible things happening.

I am still hearing stories, things they kept from me to not hurt my feelings. Laura told me recently that during her whole sixth-grade year, she was called the "AIDS girl" at school. I'd never ever heard that before.

Recently, I asked each one of our kids what they remember about that day in Duncan Gardens. I was surprised at how little they remembered the actual words Scott said. Ryan remembers lying in the grass and walking between the flowers having some conversations with his dad. Laura remembers feeling sad and confused and not saying a word on the car ride home.

Teresa asked medical questions in an attempt to stay in control, trying to keep it together. She felt like an adult when Scott told her and thought, "I can handle this; I can help take care of my sister and brother."

Scott said he, too, remembers talking to her as if she were an adult. Teresa was ten. She was ten years old.

When I think of the role that Teresa took on in trying to be good and helpful as the oldest child, trying to be an "adult," trying to be there for Laura and Ryan as her mom was sick ... all I can say is that she was a kid doing all she could, but no child should be put in that role. A fifth grader doesn't know how to digest watching her friend's sister and mom die, especially in light of the fact that her mom could die next. Yes, we were lucky, I didn't die, and their Uncle Chris didn't die either, but to grow up with that uncertainty is a lot for a child to handle.

Within the stories of tragedy and scars are stories of triumph, resilience, and overcoming. Several kids who survived being infected or affected by AIDS have grown into some of the strongest people I know. Dale has been resilient through so many obstacles and now, in his thirties, is an amazing dad to his teenage son.

My friend Tranisha was infected with HIV when she was born and beat the odds, surviving into adulthood. Tranisha lost her mother, brother, and grandmother; she ended up having to live in multiple places and a variety of situations growing up. She wrote an incredible poem that is a summary of her thoughts and feelings, her journey as a child living through the horrors and uncertainty of AIDS. Her poem ends with this:

HIV, you are just a part of me even as you're wrapped up in me.
I am still somebody with you or without you.
I want to grow to learn about who I really am and I think I am ready to move forward with you if you're gonna stay.
You have to know some things before I can forgive you but never forget
I will live a fulfilled and joyous life.
I am stronger than you now.
My family was strong too.
I deserve all the good things that come my way without you causing me any more pain.
Yes, you took a lot from me, especially in my formative years.
People you thought belonged to you but it stops with me.
This cycle of you ends with me.
I am not yours.
My family loved me, and I loved them and you can't take that from us.
HIV you lived and thrived with my family, but I don't feel so hopeless and alone anymore.

Tranisha Darlene Arzah, June 4, 2019

CONSTRUCTION
FOR CHANGE

Act as if what you do makes a difference. It does.

William James

Some things in life you just sort of fall into. My work with Construction for Change started like that. I had never once thought about working in construction nor did I have any experience or expertise in the field. But then a series of events happened that led me to CfC's door.

I first heard about this construction nonprofit from Jenny and Jason Koenig. Jenny had been Teresa's roommate in college and was one of her dearest friends. Her husband, Jason, an extremely talented director and photographer, had gone on a couple of international trips with Construction for Change to photograph CfC's work and create visual documentation of the communities they served. These photos were arranged into a gallery and displayed at the annual CfC fundraiser. Scott and I were invited by Jenny to the event and were drawn to the impact of their work.

Construction for Change has the mission of building infrastructure for other nonprofits and government agencies in impoverished communities around the world. Their purpose is to manage construction projects that increase the outreach, capacity, and care of an organization without having critical community services delayed during the construction process. Most organizations working on behalf of the poor are not experts in construction and often experience major distractions and disruptions trying to increase and maximize their community spaces. CfC aims to minimize those disruptions.

I was impressed with CfC and could see that they were filling a gap in international development. At the time, I didn't see myself being more involved than donating at their yearly fundraiser. Jason and Jenny, however, were very involved, and their photo gallery at the event was the highlight for me.

A while later, I was in my small group mentoring college students, and I started complaining about my current volunteer job with a large local nonprofit. I said, "I wish I could just work with a tiny nonprofit that does great things. One where there are fewer hoops to jump through and less paperwork. An organization where if someone has a good idea, they can just go for it."

One of the girls replied, "My brother-in-law runs an organization like that. It's called Construction for Change. His name is Nick Tosti."

A few days later I got a call from Nick Tosti.

Nick assured me that I was needed at Construction for Change. He told me that he would teach me everything I needed to know about construction and that, rest assured, I would never have to build anything. What he needed was someone to read the applications coming from organizations that needed infrastructure, then research and vet each organization to make sure they were a good fit for CfC. They needed to have the capacity to sustain their work while also caring for the newly constructed buildings, which would last for a long time. I told him I would consider the position.

At the time, Teresa and her husband, Patrick, were out of

the country. I mention this because it was a time in Jenny's life when she had more availability because some of her best friends, like Teresa, weren't around. I knew she loved CfC and I didn't want to do this potential job alone, so I asked her if she wanted to do it with me. She said, "Yes!"

I am so glad that Nick called me, and that Jenny said yes to being my partner. For three years we served as volunteer staff on what we called the Global Partnership Development Team. We read applications from organizations who wanted to partner with CfC, vetted them, and recommended to the CfC staff and Board of Directors which of the organizations we thought would make the best partners.

Jenny and I received applications from wonderful people all over the world who were doing all kinds of life-changing work on behalf of the poor. During that time, we selected several worthy projects for the CfC Board to approve, including a hospital in a remote area of Northern India; a school in the Solomon Islands, replacing one that was unsafe from wood rot, and increasing classroom space for all of the students; a medical clinic in Western Kenya; and even a couple of local Seattle projects, refurbishing a food bank and a youth center and shelter. We came to understand how a building could increase an organization's capacity, effectiveness, and outreach. It was definitely fulfilling and inspiring work.

I absolutely loved working with Nick and the whole CfC team, but I especially enjoyed working with Jenny Koenig. At the time, Laura was living in Japan and Teresa in Ireland; I missed them immensely. Not only did Jenny prove to be a more than competent team member, but she became a valued and trusted friend. She was and still is part of my extended family and, in those few years, was my "third daughter."

I learned many lessons from Jenny but perhaps none

as important as the value of showing up. One day she told me that our contribution to the world was that we were available. She added that it was our privilege that even allowed us to be available so we should take it seriously. Since that time, I have seen Jenny and her husband, Jason, take care of a friend with cancer, even driving across the United States to move their friend. I've seen them take in young friends in need, sharing their house with numerous people in various times of transition. In the middle of the isolation of COVID-19, Jenny and Jason lived in LA with a friend whose husband had died recently of a brain tumor. They provided her and her daughter with an isolation community, helping with childcare and assisting their friend with her flourishing business.

Eventually, my friendship with Jenny and my involvement with CfC led me down a path of change. My old life as an HIV advocate and public speaker was about to be awakened. My "gap year" was coming to an end.

BASEMENT

Great things are done by a series of small things
brought together.

Vincent Van Gogh

We ended up buying Sharon's rental house in North Seattle and sixteen-year-old Ryan took over the basement, creating music in his bedroom. Although those beats and melodies rattled the floor upstairs, it was fairly soundproof to the surrounding neighbors. As a high school student, he spent hours in the basement mixing music, playing guitar, editing artist photos, and, at one point, even taught guitar lessons to a junior high kid a couple of times a week.

A couple of years after moving in, Ryan moved his bedroom to the basement utility room, affectionately known as "Harry Potter's Room" under the stairs, allowing him to create a recording studio space in his old bedroom.

In 2008, when Scott and I had moved to the East Coast, Ryan was in college at the University of Washington and was working on an album with an artist from Rhode Island named Symmetry. It was at this time that his friend Ben Haggerty (Macklemore) began to hang out in the basement with Ryan for hours, recording beats and songs, which turned into an EP and then eventually turned into their music partnership,

Macklemore and Ryan Lewis. They wrote and recorded the first versions of "And We Danced," "Otherside," "Irish Celebration," "Vipassana," "The End," "Life is Cinema," "A Wake," "White Walls," and "Can't Hold Us" in that basement.

Our house in Seattle affectionately became known as The Shire. That cozy little house engulfed by an overgrown English garden has been home over the years to fifteen people and a few dogs and cats. Now and then I ask myself what if we had just driven by that day instead of going to the open house? What if Scott had toured the house with us instead of holding back and having his conversation with Sharon, the owner? What if Sharon had ignored the urge to find us and did not offer us a rental agreement we couldn't pass up? There are so many small details that could have changed the narrative of our lives, small things that led to the direction things would go, and paths that could have led a different way.

Several times, we almost bought other houses all over the city. I wonder who Ryan would've become if we had lived somewhere else. We looked at houses forty miles south, in other cities, when we moved to the Seattle area. If we had moved elsewhere, would Ryan have met his wife, Jackie, who was also a student at Roosevelt High School? Would their daughters Ramona and Ruby exist?

I'm sure everyone has thought this way with major decisions in their life. Some people would call this luck, but in my life, I have been more than nudged, almost pushed into some major life decisions that have resulted in changes or new directions in the narrative of my life. I do believe that God has something to do with our paths and I listen to those nudges.

As I write this, we are still living in that little house that we "temporarily" moved into; our basement reminds me daily that the music and films Ryan produces came out of his utmost love of creating art and would have come out one way or another, but part of that beginning was in the basement in our home in North Seattle.

TEN THOUSAND HOURS

Ten thousand hours felt like ten thousand hands,
Ten thousand hands, they carry me.

Macklemore and Ryan Lewis

O ver the years I've been told on numerous occasions that people are impressed with how independent Ryan is. These comments instantly transport me back to the dark apartment in Spokane, and I see the tiny, toddler-sized Ryan splashing milk on his cereal as I watch helplessly from the couch, too sick to move. I'm equally proud and pained hearing comments about Ryan's self-sufficiency, internalizing thoughts of failing as a parent. But more and more I'm also aware that, in his case, his independent drive has served him well. Having an internal drive that perseveres is a bonus for an artist, especially when trying to make a way into the music industry.

Around the time that Jenny and I started volunteering at CfC, Macklemore and Ryan Lewis started taking off. Ben and Ryan rented another space in North Seattle and created the studio where their Grammy Award-winning album, The Heist, would be produced. I never dreamed that I would watch from backstage as my son performed on Saturday Night Live, or watch the ball drop from the side stage as he performed in Times Square on New Year's Eve. None of this could be predicted. Our lives took an unprecedented turn when Ryan became a famous producer in what did take "10,000 hours" and a ton of hard work, yet at the same time, seemed to happen overnight.

But, again, my role was always just being Ryan's mom. People have asked me constantly since that time … "What is it like to have a famous son?"

It's like being a famous person's mom. Which, not surprisingly, is pretty similar to being a non-famous person's mom. I don't look at Ryan and think, "There's my famous child." No, I look at him and think, "There's one of my awesome kids." We may talk about different things because of the work Ryan does but we don't talk about those things any differently than if he had become an exceptional teacher or a chemist or had a passion and drive for any other profession.

I have awesome children. It is my most treasured part of surviving HIV for over thirty years that I can now have these phenomenal adult relationships with my three kids and watch them be spouses and parents.

I love Ryan. I admire him for much more than his success in music. I admire his stamina, his willingness to work on his inner life, his giving and generous spirit, his spontaneous love, and the joy he has about life in general. I love seeing him as a husband and a dad.

Ryan and I share the burden of living life in our head; we have a hard time turning off our minds and finding rest. It's what gives us each vision and ideas, and it also makes sleeping at night difficult. I have found so much grace, inspiration, and encouragement from our honest conversations about this; Ryan is often the one who helps me to keep going, keep trying, and keep moving forward.

Yes, I have a famous son. But to me, he would be a treasure even if no one else knew him. I am glad I get to share little pieces of him with the world because he has so many beautiful qualities to offer. The one thing I want you to know is that he is so much more than Macklemore and Ryan Lewis.

When I look at other famous people now, I think I see them a little differently. I see them as famous but also as people who have many layers to their lives that we, as fans, will hopefully never see. They deserve to have that privacy. They deserve to have moms who know them as their children and wives who know them as their husbands and sisters who know them as their brothers. Not their famous brother, just as their brother.

Ryan has done an amazing job of keeping himself and the rest of us grounded. He would say that at our dinner table, everyone is equally special, equally loved, and equally valued.

Except for the grandkids who steal the limelight.

GRAMMY WEDDING

A certificate on paper
Isn't gonna solve it all,
but it's a damn good place to start
No law's gonna change us
We have to change us
Whatever God you believe in
We come from the same one
Strip away the fear
Underneath it's all the same love
About time that we raised up and said so.

Macklemore and Ryan Lewis with Mary Lambert, "Same Love"

The guest list for Laura and Alex's wedding included:

Beyonce and Jay-Z
Katy Perry
Ed Sheeran
Taylor Swift
Keith Urban and Nicole Kidman
Pharrell
Bob Saget
LL Cool J
Pink
Ariana Grande
Daft Punk
Zendaya

Bruno Mars
Lady Gaga
Paul McCartney
Smokey Robinson
Ringo Starr
Yoko Ono
Steven Tyler
Stevie Wonder
Rihanna
Lorde
Alan Thicke

I suppose they wouldn't all have come if it had been a more private affair, but Laura and her fiancé, Alex, were one of thirty-three couples who were married by Queen Latifah in the middle of the 2014 Grammy Awards!

The previous December, the same day Laura went into labor with their first child, Rory, I was at the hospital awaiting his arrival when the Grammy nominations were announced, and Ryan's album with Macklemore, *The Heist*, was nominated for seven Grammy awards! To say it was an exciting time for our family would be an understatement. We were overjoyed, and Scott and I were so proud of all of our kids and the lives they were making for themselves.

In the weeks leading up to the Grammys, Ben and Ryan were asked to perform their anthem "Same Love" as a part of the Grammy ceremony on January 26, 2014. Then, just a week before the Grammys, Ryan called Laura asking her if she and Alex, who were planning on getting married that coming summer, wanted to change their plans and move their wedding up. The "Same Love" performance had evolved into an actual live group wedding that would celebrate the love and commitment of a wide variety of couples from across the US. Ryan thought it would be especially meaningful if his sister and future brother-in-law were included. Laura and Alex considered it and pretty quickly, despite having a six-week-old baby, said, "Yes!"

At that point, being that Scott and I were the only family who had originally planned to go watch the show, things kicked into high gear for us. We now needed to get Laura, Alex, and baby Rory there, as well as Teresa, Patrick, and their son, Mylo, who was six months old at the time. To make it all work we also bought a ticket for Teresa's nanny to tag along for added hands and childcare. Within forty-eight hours, Laura ran to Nordstrom with Teresa and Jackie, Ryan's wife, and thankfully was able to buy a Nicole Miller dress off the rack that she loved. Rings were purchased and all of us headed to Los Angeles.

Upon arrival, both vans headed directly to the LA County Courthouse, some of us watching sleeping babies in the van while Laura and Alex sprinted in to get a last-minute marriage license.

Everyone involved with the "Same Love" wedding— from those performing on stage (which included a choir!) to all thirty-three of the couples participating—had to do a rehearsal the day before. I was the designated babysitter and got to sit backstage with Rory during the rehearsal.

The Staples Center was abuzz the day before the Grammys. The mazes of hallways, and everything from locker rooms to spare broom closets, seemed to be turned into dressing rooms for everyone performing. Navigating the corridors was an experience, both in trying to not get lost and in trying to covertly check out what was going on. I tried not to stare or be awkward as we passed Jay-Z holding his daughter, Blue Ivy, casually having a conversation in a hallway, and Imagine Dragons heading to their sound check.

On the day of the Grammys, Laura and Alex shared a tiny

dressing room with some of the "Same Love" performers. After getting them out the door—dress steamed by Scott—rings in hand and a last-minute bouquet, I realized I wasn't feeling stressed at all about the wedding. I felt a little like Cinderella in my long gown, hair and nails done, shiny makeup, and blood-red lips! Scott, Teresa, Patrick, and I joined the masses of decked-out attendees only to find that the only venue around us serving food in the arena was ... drumroll ... McDonald's. Yes, you read that right. I went to the Grammys and ate chicken nuggets. In fact, the four of us had been so busy all day that those Big Macs, fries, and nuggets tasted amazing. And it was the first of many moments that night where I can assure you that things sure look a lot more glamorous on TV than they are when you're experiencing them.

When the Grammy ceremony started, Scott and I were in our seats way up high in the Staples Center. Our seats weren't close, but it was still a thrill to be there. Since we'd gotten some of our tickets at the last minute, our family was split up. Teresa and Patrick were sitting on the opposite side of the arena from us, next to Lorde's family, who had traveled from New Zealand. Beyonce and Jay-Z opened the show, and after their performance took seats in the front row. From where I was sitting, I could see that even Beyonce in the front row didn't have a great view of the show! She had a cameraman positioned in front of her the whole time, where he was able to easily whip between shooting the stage and shooting the reactions of her and the other celebrities around her. People at home have a better view than Beyonce!

I was excited for Laura and Alex, but had a bit of nerves for Ryan performing, as I always did, wanting things to go perfectly, especially with so many people watching. The performance/wedding, which had been kept under wraps beforehand, was a huge hit! Queen Latifah officiated, and Madonna joined Mary Lambert to sing "Same Love," which then transitioned into a beautiful moment of Madonna's "Open Your Heart" at the end of the ceremony. The newlywed couples danced in the aisles and many audience members sang along and danced in their seats. Laura and Alex were right next to Keith Urban during the ceremony; Laura reported that Keith teared up a bit watching everything and even leaned over to give them hugs as they exited. Many in the audience were visibly moved by the ceremony; no one knew they'd be attending the weddings of so many couples that night. You could feel the love, joy, and happiness.

The after-party felt like a mini reception with family and friends who'd attended the event. Since we'd been so far away during the ceremony, it was wonderful to hug and congratulate Laura and Alex—and Ryan. He did win four Grammys that night!

Asking Laura about it now, she'll tell you that the reason they jumped at this, despite being exhausted new parents, was that they recognized what an honor it would be to stand with so many different couples, some of whom were gay and had come from states where they still couldn't have legally been married in 2014. Laura is quick to point out that before 1967 and the Supreme Court's landmark "Loving Case" legalizing interracial marriage, she and Alex couldn't have been married in some states either.

After the event, I read comments from critics and conservative outlets condemning an eight-minute wedding, many saying these commitments would never last. Eight years later, I'm happy to report that Alex and Laura are going strong, as are most of the couples that they made friends with that night.

The bottom line is ... Love is love.

THE 30/30 PROJECT

At any given moment you have the power to say:
This is not how the story is going to end.

Christine Mason Miller

A round a year before my 30th anniversary of surviving HIV, March of 2014, my kids started asking me what we should do to celebrate this milestone. It was an awkward question. The idea of celebrating survival felt somewhat wrong being that so many of my friends had died of AIDS. I decided that if we could find a "pay it forward" way to observe the occasion, maybe a project that did something good for someone else in honor of our friends who had died, then I would be excited to "celebrate" in that way.

I'd been working with Construction for Change for about three years at that point. One night I was with Jenny at a CfC event at Microsoft, watching a slideshow presentation by one of our project managers. The photos were of a hospital that had been built in Northern India. Even though, as volunteer staff at Construction for Change, I'd helped set up this project, and for the past year, read weekly updates about the hospital being built, until I saw the photos, I didn't know that this hospital was built almost entirely by women.

There they were, women in their saris, their long Indian dresses with cement bags on their heads and tools in their hands, building a hospital. Martha, the project manager, went on to explain that although CfC pays a fair wage, these women were not motivated to build the hospital because of money or income. They were building a hospital because they were tired of their children dying in transport to the nearest medical facility, hours and hours away, many times only getting there to be turned away at the door because they were poor and could not pay.

I looked sideways at Jenny during that slideshow and said, "Wow! Those women built a freaking hospital."

I was struck and amazed by these determined moms. *They* were my seed, my spark, and the beginning of the idea of the 30/30 Project. I wanted to provide healthcare to people who didn't have access, like the women in India had done.

As a public health advocate, I strongly believe that a person's health should not be determined by where they live or by how much money they have.

I, myself, had survived some difficulties in the healthcare system living with HIV. Although these were unpleasant experiences for me, compared to stories I would hear regarding lack of healthcare access and discrimination for the world's extreme poor, mine were mere stories of ignorance and inconvenience. At the end of the day, I had doctors, I had medications, I had health insurance, I had money to pay for my healthcare bills, and I had a car to drive to those appointments.

Never did I fear that my child would die because I couldn't get to a doctor's office, and never in my wildest dreams could I imagine being turned away with my sick child at the door of a clinic or hospital because I couldn't pay.

I began to think about the idea of our family raising money and donating it to CfC to build a clinic for a health-serving nonprofit working in an area where the incidence of HIV infection was high and access to comprehensive healthcare was low. I began to write letters to organizations that were providing excellent healthcare in under-resourced communities around the world and asked if they knew of any community that needed a building or infrastructure to increase their capacity, outreach, and care.

I got a few responses, but by far the most compelling was from the Boston-based nonprofit, Partners In Health.

Years earlier, I'd read Tracy Kidder's book *Mountains Beyond Mountains* about Paul Farmer and was in awe of the healthcare delivery he'd established and developed in Haiti among rural impoverished communities. I loved his mantra that all people deserve quality healthcare. Dr. Farmer began his work in Haiti while he was still in medical school at Harvard and went on to be the founder of Partners In Health in 1987, taking his high standard of healthcare into the poorest parts of the world and offering those services for free. Farmer believed that no one should die of preventable disease. He believed that healthcare was a human right, along with clean water, food, education, and shelter.

I went after PIH. I asked them to apply to partner with us. I said to them, "Please don't send me a project you're going to build anyway. Send me something that won't happen, a health center that won't get built unless we help you build it."

They sent me three proposals, and one was to build a primary health clinic in the Neno District of Malawi, a place of extreme poverty where the nearest healthcare facility was a two-hour drive on a good day, where precarious dirt roads could make the trek even longer. I use the word "drive" loosely because almost all of the people living in that area did not own cars.

PIH had been taking mobile clinics into the Neno District for some time, but there was a desperate need for a health center to be open on a daily basis, serving the twenty thousand people living in that area of Malawi, a country where one in ten adults were infected with HIV. Not only was I excited to bring lifesaving medications and treatment to a place that had fewer healthcare options than I did in 1990, but also, as an HIV prevention specialist, it didn't escape me that the health education coming from this clinic would also prevent countless new infections and eventually lower the HIV rate in the region.

I was enthusiastic about this idea to build in Neno, so I decided to take the proposal to my family and see what they thought.

When I first told Ryan, "I have an idea: let's build a clinic in Malawi for Partners In Health," I thought he would remember Paul Farmer from the only health book I ever remember him reading, *Mountains Beyond Mountains*. At the time he'd concluded that Paul was the real-life "House," his favorite fictional doctor on TV.

Instead, he said, "What's Partners In Health?"

It didn't take long to connect the dots between Farmer, the book, and PIH, but what came out of Ryan's mouth next was the biggest surprise. He replied, "Mom, we can't build just one clinic. You've lived thirty years—we need to build thirty healthcare buildings."

Thirty clinics or healthcare buildings are definitely more than one. Way more than one.

I'm not sure how Ryan and the rest of the family talked me into saying yes, but within a short amount of time we were planning an Indiegogo crowdfunding campaign to build thirty healthcare buildings.

I originally called our project the 30 for 30, thirty buildings for thirty years. Before we launched the Indiegogo, we abruptly changed the name to the 30/30 Project because ESPN simultaneously launched a show called *30 for 30*.

The project now had a name, and the ball was rolling.

Next, I asked Shelby Stoner, the Executive Director for Construction for Change, if they would allow our project to be umbrellaed under the CfC brand. If so, if we set up a joint initiative between our family and this construction management nonprofit, we felt that there was no reason to become our own nonprofit. The idea was that we would vet the projects and raise funds to build the thirty facilities while CfC would manage the design and construction.

Here's the thing: right then and there Shelby or the CfC Board could have just said, "No."

"No, this is a bad, risky idea. Not the direction we want to go."

And that would've been it. There may have never been a 30/30 Project.

But they didn't say no. They said, "Yes."

So here we were in April 2014. Ryan, me, Shelby, and Ryan's manager Zach huddled together at Ryan's studio trying to come up with a plan to make the 30/30 Project happen. In the space of a week, we built a website and gathered perks for the campaign, including T-shirts that said Healthcare Is A Human Right on one side and 30/30 Project on the other.

Ryan created a very compelling launch video for our three-week Indiegogo campaign. It's still on YouTube and has almost four hundred thousand views. When I was being interviewed for the video, I was so nervous; my confidence in public speaking did not transfer to being filmed.

Ryan being Ryan worked magic with cutting, editing, photo overlays, and B-roll. When asked about the reasoning behind the project, I said, "I want to do something big. The 30/30 Project is that big idea. We believe that healthcare is a human right. We have the knowledge, and we have the treatments. Life-threatening diseases like HIV/AIDS can be managed. What people need is access."

The day I finally got to see the completed film, tears streamed down my face when Ryan started by saying, "I want to tell you about the strongest woman I know: my mom, Julie Lewis."

Dang.

I was deeply touched, and my heart was full. I also began to feel very responsible to have this effort be successful, to make my family proud. Little did I know at the moment that my quest for success and fear of failure would haunt me for the next five years.

We launched the 30/30 Project on April 22, 2014. Our goal was to raise funds to build thirty healthcare projects around the world in areas that lacked healthcare access, and we were on a deadline to complete the funding in five years.

On launch day, we were featured on *CBS This Morning*. Ryan and I were interviewed in his studio on the waterfront in downtown Seattle by Ben Tracy and a news team from CBS.

In the feature they ended up using a lot of footage from Ryan's launch video along with some family pictures intermixed with our interview, explaining why we were doing the project and, because Ryan was the celebrity, focusing quite a bit on his life.

Ben Tracy asked Ryan, "What do you remember as a child growing up with a mom who had HIV?"

"I remember periods of fear as a child," said Ryan.

"Did you ever think that at some point with your success that this would come out to the public?"

"Well," Ryan replied, "I have an AIDS ribbon tattoo on my arm." He showed the tattoo that winds from his wrist to his elbow. "If you do that, you have to be ready to talk about it."

He asked me if this was just about celebrating my survival, and I answered, "This is also about our friends who died of AIDS; there is survivor guilt there. I want to do something to honor all those people who we dearly loved, who died along the way."

The documentary went on to say that our goal was to build thirty healthcare centers serving six hundred thousand people.

Then he asked Ryan a great question. "If you weren't Ryan Lewis, of Macklemore and Ryan Lewis, is this possible?" Adding, "Could you do this?"

"I don't think you would be here," Ryan said.

And then simultaneously we all kind of chuckled, and both of them said under their breath, "That's probably true."

Ryan then added, "It's pretty amazing for me that my family could have this story, my mom could go through all of this, and it could come to this point. That I could use the platform that has been provided to invest my time and energy into something that is really positive."

Ben Tracy ended the interview with this: "It's a way to honor life's unexpected gifts, not sudden fame, but a mom you never expected to live to see it."

Exactly.

They ended the segment by saying that Ryan, Ben Haggerty, and his wife, Tricia Davis, were the first donors to the 30/30 Project. For me, the proudest moment as a mom was when Gayle King said that she respected Ryan for using his celebrity platform to give back. I was proud, but, again, I also felt a deep sense of personal responsibility that I needed to fulfill the promises we were making. It felt like now, after sharing our plan with America, Ryan's reputation was on the line as well.

In the following three weeks, Indiegogo donations poured in from everywhere. We received funds from people I hadn't seen in years, notes from people I worked with at the health department in Spokane, high school and college friends, and people on my old speakers' bureau. Some of my HIV-positive women friends posted a photo on Facebook, wishing us luck and saying how proud they were of me. I was extremely touched when I saw it.

The level of generosity and love was over the top. The majority of notes and donations were from strangers. People were so encouraging. Ryan, Shelby, and I read almost everything that came our way.

Many of the emails and letters were from people whose parents or relatives had died or were living with HIV along with mail from young adults who were infected with HIV themselves. We made it a priority to try to answer most of those emails and letters. The thing was, Ryan and I related to all of the stories people shared because we weren't in any way famous or known when our family was struggling with AIDS at our home in Spokane in the 1990s; we were just an average family dealing with an unexpected disease. We saw ourselves in those letters and emails.

The campaign was followed by a whirlwind of public appearances. We were guests on *Anderson Cooper 360*, Elvis Duran's *Morning Show*, and we had features in *People Magazine* and *Rolling Stone*. To say it was overwhelming for me would be an understatement. Ryan was used to the media world and helped me through each interview, but I was nervous and a bit awkward every time.

Those first couple of weeks we funded three clinics through the campaign and shortly after had two other donors each commit to pay for a clinic. In a very short time, five clinics had funding and plans to be built. We had selected the healthcare partners we would build for in advance; those first five projects were in Malawi, Uganda, India, and two in Kenya.

The 30/30 Project was now in motion and real communities with real people needing healthcare were counting on us. I felt responsible for the well-being of many people.

THE LONG GAME

He who would learn to fly one day
must first learn to stand and walk and run
and climb and dance;
one cannot fly into flying.

Nietzsche

After the initial campaign finished, and all the buzz began to settle, the 30/30 Project became yesterday's news and Ryan went back to doing what he does best, making music. Shelby had CfC to run and went back to focusing on her already-full schedule.

I clearly remember waking up in the middle of the night, alone, thinking to myself, "Holy shit! What in the world did I just tell all of America that I was going to do?" I was a bit terrified. The task seemed impossible and overwhelming.

Looking back, I have to thank Ryan for stretching me. For having a bigger vision than I would have ever had, one that kept me awake at night and, to be honest, made me terribly uncomfortable. I would have never jumped into that pool, the bottomless thirty-healthcare-facilities pool that is. I'd needed to be pushed.

What did the next several months feel like? Fundraising was hard work. I knew it would be because Scott had spent a good portion of his career in nonprofit development. Raising money for an organization or project was hard even when that nonprofit had great programs and was doing tremendous work. But procuring funds was even harder when your project hadn't really done anything yet. I was asking donors to buy into and support an idea, a plan.

That first year, after the initial boom of the Indiegogo campaign, raising money for the 30/30 Project was slow going. I spoke to anyone and everyone, and gave speeches at any event that would have me, sharing our vision of healthcare as a human right and the idea that infrastructure could increase access to healthcare for the world's most vulnerable people.

I was tired; don't forget, I have AIDS. I wasn't at all sure how we would ever make our five-year goal to fund the thirty projects. Then, toward the end of that first year, we were fortunate to hire my daughter, Teresa, to be the director of the 30/30 Project. Teresa had been working at Swedish Medical Center; her job experience along with her degree in International Studies made her more than qualified to lead us.

I said to Teresa one day right after she was hired, "Do you think people will think badly of us if we only build fifteen healthcare centers?"

I mean, we were not, at that point, hitting our targets to finish in five years. It was a real question. Would anything short of thirty feel like we had failed?

That decision, hiring Teresa, was the turning point toward the success and progress the 30/30 Project experienced. Being a strong strategic planner, Teresa mapped out a road for success, she hired very capable consultants, and then blew them all away by outpacing their furthest projections of what the 30/30 Project could do and how quickly we could do it. In short, after Teresa began to steer our boat, things progressed at a faster and more efficient rate.

I know for a fact that we could not and would not have completed this endeavor in five years without her.

MORE THAN A BUILDING

A building is not just a place to be but a way to be.

Frank Lloyd Wright

In the summer of 2015, after a year and a half of partnering on projects and raising funds, the 30/30 team traveled to Kenya to visit some of the completed buildings. Leaving Nairobi, we started out in a van driving on freeways and then, gradually, side road after side road, which led us to a winding dirt road in the beautiful agricultural community of Kangundo, Kenya.

I'd spent the last six months getting weekly updates and photos of this clinic being built from our partner organization, Kizimani, but no photo compares with actually seeing the real-life building in context. What caught my attention as we drove up were the soccer field next to the beautiful new clinic and the school on the other side of the field, neither of which were evident in photos. The clinic was situated in a great location, especially for parents and their kids.

The sight of the new building was incredible, but what I experienced next is hard to describe. Miriam Won, one of the directors of Kizimani, had said to me many times, "This clinic at Kizimani—it's much more than a building."

After touring the clinic, we were instructed to go up the hill where we would have a surprise from the community.

Women in brightly colored dresses greeted us with singing and dancing. I jumped out of the van as soon as I could and was drawn into the festivities, awkwardly dancing but mostly just smiling and hugging everyone who was welcoming us. Next, a delicious meal appeared and more singing. The most memorable part of the day came when we circled around and started sharing.

I was aware that many of the women and men at Kizimani were HIV-positive, but they did not know my story, so I took some time to share why I wanted to build healthcare facilities, including my own history as a woman living with AIDS. My honesty opened a pandora's box of sorts with one person after another telling their own stories and sharing what this clinic meant to them.

It's hard to put into words how impactful that day was for me. I heard stories of gratitude from people for whom healthcare services were now available within walking distance of their rural homes; I also began to hear of other changes that were happening because of the new building.

I listened to accounts of men and women who were employed during the construction of the clinic, in an area where jobs were hard to come by. People who'd been trained in new methods of construction could now take those new skills and get other employment. Then there were the groundskeepers who had helped with the construction and now had jobs maintaining the clinic. The facility was rippling out to affect lives in ways beyond delivering healthcare.

In some of our completed projects, that ripple has even gone further as new businesses crop up around the healthcare buildings because they are places where community members gather. Often new jobs create enough income for families so kids can now attend school because their parents can pay school fees. Sometimes the new building is the only one in the community with electricity. Many are used by students at night to study because they are the only ones with light. One of our clinics ran a line from their generator under a highway to the neighboring school so that the school would have light. These are just some of the ripple effects of building in remote, rural, impoverished communities. This is in addition to the new healthcare access, treatment and prevention available to community members.

The stories I heard at Kizimani were all filled with hope and gratitude. We had to leave far too soon to beat the Nairobi rush hour, and as we drove away, some women in the community were making soap to sell at the local market. They said they'd figured out a formula to make the best soap in town, and after spending the day with them, I'm sure this was true.

I left admiring the resourcefulness, generosity, creativity, and great faith of the wonderful people of Kangundo. Being in Kenya confirmed the original vision of the 30/30 Project, of actively searching for building partners and projects that are community led, owned, and operated.

I saw firsthand that access to quality healthcare not only created healthier individuals but also, collectively, healthier communities.

HIV PREVENTION

Measure what is measurable,
and make measurable what is not so.

Galileo Galilei

had just returned from Kizimani where I met many people who were now receiving access to comprehensive healthcare. I'd heard their stories and suddenly what had been transactional for me became much more relational. Simple numbers on a page didn't convey the difference that HIV prevention was making on a practical, everyday level in people's lives who were receiving care. It made me think even more about how important it is to keep people from being infected with HIV in the first place.

Solving inequalities in healthcare has often been transactional. We boil it down to tasks, things to do, and programs that ensure progress, providing more access to treatment and prevention.

We don't measure prevention in the moments of a life that can now be lived. What does it mean when a parent doesn't die, when a baby is born healthy, or when a life is lengthened?

Asking these questions brought to my mind lyrics from the song "Seasons of Love," from *Rent*, one of my favorite musicals. The song asks the heartfelt question ... "How do you measure a year in a life ... How do you measure the life of a woman or a man?"

How can we, as the song points out, measure in love? Disease prevention is important not just because of what it stops but because of what it enables. What HIV prevention allows are the moments that would have been lost, the journeys that can now be traveled, and the lives that can now be shared. While visiting Kizimani, I met a man who had quit his job to care for his wife while she died of AIDS. His lack of income resulted in his two children dropping out of school because he could not pay the fees.

Access to healthcare and HIV prevention might have prevented her death and the devastating ripple effect on his family.

I also met an HIV-positive new mother who had a happier story. She was fortunate to receive prenatal care and medication that prevents transmission of the virus to her newborn girl. Her hope is to stay healthy, despite her diagnosis, by taking lifesaving medications. She can now see her child grow up and even someday, perhaps, become a grandmother like me.

For this woman, HIV prevention and treatment wasn't about statistics, it was about time. Time to be a parent or grandparent, a sister, a spouse, lover, friend, or co-worker. Time to laugh, cry, create, screw up, hang out, contribute, and love. Time to live. HIV prevention was a gift of time.

When we lose someone close to us, we don't necessarily miss them because of the things they could have accomplished. Really, we miss them because of the hole they leave in our lives when they're gone. I often recall memories of my friends who died of AIDS and I wonder, "What would Joyce, Kara, Camie, Mary, George, Barry, Craig, Mark, and

Harold have done if they had been given the gift of time? Whose lives didn't get enriched and blessed because they missed out on spending time and receiving love from these wonderful people who died years ago?"

The man I met in Kenya doesn't miss his wife because of what she might've done; he misses her because he and his children loved her and miss the love they received from her now that she's gone.

HIV prevention is not only a gift of time; HIV prevention is also a gift of love.

MANDELAS

I carry with me the values of my grandfather.
I am an African and I know what it means
to be African—and I'm proud of it.

Ndaba Mandela

I met Nelson Mandela's grandson, Kweku Mandela, several years ago when he was visiting Seattle and came by Ryan's studio to meet the Macklemore team. This began a relationship with not only Kweku, but also his cousin Ndaba Mandela. Both of these men continue their grandfather's legacy through their lives, their international work, and their outreach to African youth. In 2010, Kweku and Ndaba founded Africa Rising Foundation, an organization dedicated to empowering young people to be at the forefront of Africa's development.

I am one of their biggest fans.

When I think about children who have had their lives upended by AIDS and yet gone on to not only survive but turn their pain into a powerful force of goodness and positive change, I think of Ndaba Mandela. AIDS caused the death of his mother, Zondi, in 2003, and the family hid the truth to avoid stigma, public scrutiny, and fear surrounding the disease in the country with the highest HIV prevalence in the world, South Africa.

Ndaba said, "I was familiar with the mental gymnastics that people practiced in order to avoid telling the truth."

When his father, Makgatho, died of AIDS in 2005, the family met to decide "what should be said" about his father's death, knowing they could just say that he died of pneumonia or tuberculosis. But Ndaba writes in his book about his grandfather that Nelson Mandela announced his family would tell the truth and not hide it; Ndaba's father had died of AIDS. "'No,' the Old Man barked, and the room fell silent. 'We will not say that. We will say that HIV/AIDS killed him. Let's stop beating around the bush. We need to fight the stigma, not facilitate it.'"

That announcement was akin to Magic Johnson's announcement in the United States years earlier, which helped to begin destigmatizing the disease and allowing more normality, discussion, and acceptance of the people who were infected. Mandela's announcement was the start of a major change in the fight to end AIDS, not only in South Africa, but around the world.

Ndaba was a young adult when his parents died. He was in his formative years, and their deaths changed the course of his life. He went on to be an ambassador for UNAIDS, dedicating his life to the eradication of HIV and empowering the next generation of youth. To mark the tenth anniversary of Africa Rising, the Mandela Institute for Humanity was established to teach young people about the leadership style and values of Nelson Mandela, including humility, discipline, resilience, and passion. Ndaba is an inspiration to me to keep going and to help build a better future.

I had the opportunity to speak alongside Ndaba for a UNAIDS event in Basel, Switzerland. The focus of the event was raising money for pediatric AIDS and the prevention of mother-to-child transmission around the globe. It was an honor to be in the lineup of amazing speakers, including Kofi Annan, the seventh Secretary-General of the United Nations. I was very jet lagged and, being that it was a gala that went into the wee hours of the night, I didn't speak until after ten. I have a thing where I try to memorize my speeches so I can maintain eye contact and rapport with my audience and that night my talk was fairly short so I figured I could just give the speech without notes.

This was the only time I have ever, mid-talk, had a complete and total block of what I was saying. That night, halfway through my address, I just stood there like a deer in headlights. For about half a minute, which seemed like an hour, I shut my eyes and I said to the audience, "I just need a second," and then, miraculously, the words came back and I went on.

To say I was disappointed in myself would be an understatement. I was embarrassed.

But then an amazing thing happened. People started coming up to me and telling me how touched they were when I got overwhelmed by emotion talking about kids and moms with AIDS.

I was like, "Oh, is that what I was doing?"

UNAIDS raised a lot of money that night, and I was told over and over that it was helpful when I spoke from the heart with so much emotion. While that is not exactly what happened, I'm delighted people chose to see and experience it differently.

I remember Basel and my "disaster" speech every time I think of Ndaba Mandela, who, by the way, delivered a flawless speech that night.

TOGO

Individually we are a drop.
Together, we are an ocean.

Ryunosuke Satoro

I first met Jennifer Schechter and was introduced to Integrate Health, an organization providing access to healthcare in Togo, West Africa, when they applied to be one of our 30/30 Projects. I have to admit that when I read the application from IH, I actually had to look up where in the world Togo was.

Since then, I witnessed Jennifer receive an award from Chelsea Clinton and the Clinton Foundation, and I watched her give several impressive presentations. But I learned that you don't really know Jennifer Schechter until you see her in Togo with the Integrate Health staff of well over one hundred people, almost all of whom are Togolese.

Jennifer is originally from New York, and she received her master's degree in social work and public health from the University of Washington, right down the street from my house. She co-founded Integrate Health and opened the first rural HIV treatment center in Togo in 2004 after her time there in the Peace Corps. She has been working to fight preventable deaths of women and children in Togo ever since.

When I read the application for Integrate Health, I was overwhelmed by the stories of healthcare disparity. Everything from delivering babies on a stone table by the light of a cell phone flashlight that was wedged between the head and neck of the midwife, to delivering in clinics that lacked electricity, had no running water, and no bathrooms. Several were infested with bats and other pests.

When I read stories about mothers who were desperate for a two-dollar pill to save their children from dying of malaria, a pill they knew existed but didn't have access to, I felt their urgency. We were thrilled to partner with women in Togo to increase the quality of healthcare options and make accessing that care closer, easier, and more comprehensive.

When we started working with Integrate Health in 2017, they were the only international organization working with the Togolese Ministry of Health to provide healthcare in Togo. They were partnering with the government in nine healthcare centers and had ninety staff members. At the time, they also had an aggressive expansion plan. We started by agreeing to renovate four health clinics and to build a brand-new maternity ward in the largest urban center in Northern Togo. Those four clinics served fifty villages and enabled ten thousand women and children to access free maternal and child healthcare services—services not offered elsewhere.

"In Togo, we aren't just a drop in the bucket ... we are THE drop in the bucket," Jennifer has said several times about Integrate Health.

Our 30/30 team, along with Ryan's wife, Jackie, and photographer Zoe Rain, had the privilege to go to Togo in January 2018 to see the five initial 30/30 Projects built there by Construction for Change: the brand-new maternity ward and four renovated health clinics in the rural Kara region. We traveled with Jennifer and met fifty community health workers that Integrate Health employs in that area. Jennifer translated everything we had to say into French with nurses, community members, and tribal chiefs.

Sometimes I'd ask her at the end of a visit with a chief, "Did you translate everything I was saying? Or, did you add in the things you were wishing I was saying that you really wanted the chief to hear?" Jennifer smiled and chuckled but never really answered my question.

Many of the local Togolese we met called Teresa "Grande-Fille" or oldest daughter while referring to Jackie as "Belle-Fille" meaning beautiful daughter. We learned that this endearing title was for the newlywed or newest daughter-in-law. We teased Jackie about this but took it to a whole other level when twice she was predicted to have a wonderful marriage blessed with twins! We laughed and pondered as we drove around Togo: "Was that a true blessing or a future curse?"

Although most of the building we undertook with the 30/30 Project was brand new construction, in Togo we decided to renovate existing structures.

When we remodel a kitchen in the US, perhaps we replace everything that is old or outdated with new stuff: new counters, new appliances, new sinks, new colors. We create a more current style, perhaps taking out the laminated counters and linoleum floors, replacing them with granite and subway tile, or maybe a new "green" product to reduce our carbon footprint.

In Togo, when we talked about renovating clinics, we weren't talking about replacing things—we were talking about adding things. Adding electricity and water access where there were none, and adding bathrooms so people didn't have to use the neighbor's field. We needed to add waiting areas, so the mothers and their children didn't have to stand outside in a line wrapped around the building, in triple-digit temperatures, for hours. Some of the clinics were infested with bats so we also needed to remove pests and mold.

I couldn't imagine taking my child to a doctor's office where there was no electricity, no water, no bathrooms, and where the medical staff had to wipe bat feces off of the counters every morning to start the day. Our whole 30/30 Project team strongly felt that the families in Togo deserved better. So much better.

While in Togo, we toured the first five completed projects, and we were happy to see that the renovations had brought lights, electricity, running water, and bathrooms. The clinics were also finally pest free—no more bats, wasps, or rodents.

The best part of the renovated clinics in Togo wasn't the buildings. The best part was the free healthcare Integrate Health offered to all pregnant women and children under five years old. One woman I talked to said, "With free healthcare at my clinic, now I don't have to wait to go to the doctor when my child gets sick."

I came to realize the whole concept of "waiting" for healthcare proved too often to be detrimental and sometimes deadly.

One afternoon, we attended a huge community celebration in our honor. Hundreds of people showed up to thank us and CfC for their new facilities. When I told one of the IH staff that I was surprised by the large turnout, he simply said, "Their babies are no longer dying. It's a big deal."

This truth hit me hard. Local and affordable access to healthcare was, literally, saving lives.

I was also reminded that the reason we were even there in the first place was because the women in Togo, especially the community health workers, had advocated for themselves and their community members to improve healthcare options in their area. I witnessed firsthand while visiting that health is highly valued in this culture. One Saturday morning, Zoe, our photographer, was out filming, and she saw a whole neighborhood on a community jog. While driving, we passed stand after stand of fresh vegetables for sale. Physical fitness and strong bodies are celebrated in Togo. The lack of healthcare options did not mean that the Togolese do not value health. They simply lacked the resources and access. Their investment and energy in improving healthcare access were evident to our staff.

In Togo, I had the opportunity to speak to a whole room of HIV-positive people, including several small children. It was humbling, to say the least. Jennifer translated everything I said into French. Despite the language barrier, I felt very close to everyone in the room; they were listening carefully to what I was sharing. Even though our lives were worlds apart, we still had some of the same struggles—I could see that in their eyes as I was talking. I'd been sick all that day, very sick—but I would have never missed this opportunity.

When I finished telling my story, there was an open time for sharing. Several in the group told me about the complications and supply chain issues they have in Togo getting HIV medicine, such as antiretrovirals. It made me remember how fortunate I have been with healthcare access, treatment, and care.

I will never experience their hardships with HIV. But one thing I do know: there can be oceans, borders, politics, and even physical walls separating people, but the shared human experience, the compassion, and the shared stories cut through all of that very quickly.

After that trip, our 30/30 team committed to rehabbing seven more clinics in Togo. While we were there, we had the opportunity to visit one of the "before" renovation clinics, to see firsthand what the buildings were like before Construction for Change and their project managers worked their magic.

If I could transport smells from that clinic into this book, that would say it all. Black mold so bad you could feel it in your throat, leaks in the ceiling, bat feces everywhere, toxic air, and bathrooms you didn't want to get within ten feet of. Two people were waiting for care in this clinic compared with full waiting rooms of thirty or more at the newly renovated healthcare centers.

It's not a wonder that Togolese mothers didn't want to take their children to these toxic clinics or risk their lives delivering their babies there. They were choosing, instead, to take another risk by delivering their babies, unattended, at home. We met these moms and kids as they waited for those clinics to get rebuilt. Integrate Health and the 30/30 Project renovations were their plan for better healthcare.

As our partnership with Integrate Health expanded, we watched as they continued to grow, now employing over two hundred community health workers. Their relationship with the Ministry of Health has expanded, even advising and supplying protective gear and safe spaces in response to the coronavirus.

Their goal is to significantly increase the number of children who make it to their fifth birthday. Integrate Health is progressively making that a reality for many kids in Togo.

OUT OF TIME

*Human beings to me are not more or less human
depending on the nation state in which they were born.
I want everyone to have access to health care.*

Dr. Joia Mukherjee

One of the first 30/30 Projects we took on was building a clinic in Western Kenya, in the city of Mbita for our healthcare partner Med25. By 2018, that clinic had been operational for some time, but they desperately needed to increase their capacity. The Med25 clinic had an excellent model of healthcare delivery and provided the Mbita community with free services, but they were lacking an overnight inpatient clinic and maternity ward, which we committed to and eventually built for them.

But for Grace, that inpatient clinic did not come soon enough.

Before the inpatient clinic was operational, Grace showed up at Med25 with her four-year-old son, Brian, who had a fever, achiness, and diarrhea. The nurse diagnosed him with severe malaria and herbal poisoning. Apparently, Grace had given him herbs at the suggestion of her mother-in-law who thought he was bewitched.

Unfortunately, Brian was so sick that he needed round-the-clock IVs and overnight monitoring of his vital signs, requiring an extended stay at an inpatient facility, which

Med25 did not have yet. So, the nurse referred Grace and Brian to the only hospital that had the IV medications he needed, thirty miles away, a hospital that would charge Grace more money than she had.

The healthcare worker from Med25 who sent us this story ended it with this:

> As I am writing a referral letter, what is running through my mind are questions.
>
> If we had inpatient wards, would I be writing this letter or administering the right medication to Brian?
>
> Would I be wasting Brian's precious time counseling his mother on the need to go to the hospital or would I be saving his life?

For Grace and Brian, it was a race against time. Life expectancy for an infant or small child with malaria decreases significantly with each hour. It's the difference between administering an oral medication or having to start IVs for a convulsing child. Time was critical.

You know, when we launched the 30/30 Project, I wanted it to be a five-year project, mostly for my own convenience. But as these buildings became reality, I realized that every day we wasted, every delay we encountered in bringing healthcare access to these communities in need, actually cost lives. Real lives.

The longer we took meant that some people weren't going to make it. Usually, it was the most vulnerable: children, pregnant moms, the elderly, and the extreme poor. Why did I want to finish these thirty healthcare buildings?

Because Brian's mom was out of options. Grace, and many other moms, were needlessly watching their kids die of preventable causes.

One healthcare worker I met called it, "Dying of the stupid diseases."

NO MOM LEFT BEHIND

Every eleven seconds, a pregnant woman
or newborn dies somewhere around the world.

UNICEF, September 2019

When Teresa was in elementary school, she loved playing the computer game "Oregon Trail." These days, Teresa, Laura, and I are quick to point out that none of us would've have survived on the real Oregon Trail. We would have all died in childbirth. After having experienced an unexpected medical emergency when I gave birth, I worried and prayed for my daughters as they experienced an emergency C-section, and a sudden, unexpected premature birth. These were traumatic experiences that they had not planned for or thought about when they prepared for childbirth. If we had been pioneer women out on the Oregon Trail, in the vast wilderness with no medical supplies, physicians, or medical clinic, our horrendous childbirth experiences would surely have prevented us from arriving in Oregon alive.

For millions around the world who live on less than two dollars a day, their chance of surviving any medical complication is much closer to that experienced on the Oregon Trail. Lack of medical access and potential death is not a game. It's a daily reality and is particularly heartbreaking when occasions that should be joyous, like the birth of a baby, become a death sentence for a new mother.

A few years into the 30/30 Project we began to get a lot of applications to build maternity wards and were confronted by the need to improve the delivery of healthcare to women and children in communities around the world. In 2016, we launched the first Mother's Day campaign to build a maternity ward and continued the campaign for the next two years for other worthy partners. We called the campaign No Mom Left Behind.

After all, I was infected with HIV in a maternity ward after hemorrhaging for twelve hours. I felt a connection to the women these buildings would serve, as did Teresa and Laura. Healthy moms and babies became a critical area of focus for the 30/30 Project. We committed to help women-serving health organizations have the best spaces to provide excellent care and improve maternal outcomes for their communities.

More than three hundred thousand women around the world die in childbirth or complications with pregnancy each year. When I think of my life with HIV, and the beginning of that being, that I had a tainted blood transfusion and then a dismal prognosis that I would die young ... I can see that even my story is a story of privilege—it is a story of doctors, medicine, hospitals, and care.

If I had been in a different place during my delivery of baby Teresa, like in a rural African countryside where 80 percent of communities lack access to healthcare, I would have died from the hemorrhage. Period. And my baby might have died, too. There would have been no blood transfusion. No AIDS story.

My story and many of our sad healthcare stories are still stories of very privileged lives.

Recently I learned that the blood bank that supplied the HIV-infected blood for my transfusion is working globally to develop innovations to improve outcomes from pregnancy-related complications due to blood loss. Their recent blog post stating that "no woman should die giving life" indicates that this is a different era where many are collaborating to solve healthcare disparities worldwide.

Unfortunately, these disparities in the quality of care for different people also exist right here in the US. Although mothers here usually fare better than women in Togo or Uganda, we still have the highest mortality rate in childbirth of any other developed nation in the world, a rate almost double most high-income countries. If that weren't a big enough discrepancy, looking at the data further shows that maternal mortality for black women is two and a half times worse than for white or Hispanic women, even when all other factors are equal.

Internally, humans are biologically the same—the uterus of a black person or white person doesn't look or function any differently—so why are our healthcare outcomes so drastically different? It's racism, classism, and not taking women seriously when they explain their pain and symptoms. Statistics are proving this over and over.

Joia Adele Crear-Perry, an OB-GYN and founder of the National Birth Equity Collaborative, said it well: "We're not biologically different; there's no Black gene or Black heart or Black kidneys. We've spent generations blaming Black people for their outcomes without really addressing the underlying root causes of racism, classism, and gender oppression. So, when people ask me what is the cause of Black maternal death, the answer is not race. It's racism."

With the right care, this doesn't have to happen, and the right care begins with a safe and welcoming space to give birth and an educated nondiscriminatory medical staff. Women sacrifice many things when they become a mother, but they shouldn't have to sacrifice their lives.

LAURA GOES TO KENYA

What are we here for if not to help each other?

Wendo Aszed, Dandelion Africa

One of my favorite trips with the 30/30 Project was in 2019 when we went back to Kenya and visited several of our finished facilities while scoping out possibilities for future buildings. What made it extra special for me was that my daughter, Laura, joined us. I had wanted to include all our family on the journey of bringing healthcare to communities around the world, and by this point the only person whose life and work had not intersected with 30/30 was Laura. I desperately wanted to take her on an international trip, and it was finally happening! HIV had been her family story, too, and I would have regretted the project ending without her insight coming forth from being directly involved.

So off we flew to Nairobi.

We started out in the Kenyan capital and then headed west by car to Kisumu to explore both the north and south regions of Western Kenya. On my first trip to Kenya, a couple of years earlier, I'd flown when traveling long distances; this time driving across the country was a totally different experience and one that gave me a new perspective. Instead of going on a safari to see zebras and warthogs, we just watched them in the wild on the side of the road from seats in our rental van.

One of the 30/30 partners we visited in Kenya was the organization Dandelion Africa, where a newly constructed maternity ward was scheduled to be opened. When it came to healthcare, rural Kenya had many of the same obstacles as Togo. We chose this organization because when we read the application and heard the raving referrals as well as the stellar report from our project manager, who visited the property on a preconstruction trip, we knew we'd found another jewel in Dandelion Africa and their Executive Director, Wendo Aszed.

Wendo Aszed grew up in the rural Rift Valley of Kenya. When she finished high school, she left her village, pursued a business degree in college, and got an excellent job in the city.

Just like me, Wendo thought that HIV only happened to other people, and it wasn't until her best friend died of AIDS that she knew she needed to do something about it. Wendo went back to her community in the Rift Valley and started visiting different villages, talking to women, and identifying the specific issues each community faced. The problems she saw led her to found Dandelion Africa eleven years ago, focusing on the most marginalized people in her community: women, girls, and youth.

When it came to healthcare, the main obstacles limiting access to women were: poverty—they could not afford the cost of care; distance—it was eleven miles to the nearest rudimentary health center; and tribal practices—child marriage, which meant most girls didn't continue their education and were often pregnant before they finished grade school, and female genital mutilation or FGM, a practice that critically changed the sexual and maternal health of the young girls who received it.

Dandelion Africa focuses on the whole person. They often say, "A healthy baby doesn't begin when a woman gets pregnant. A healthy baby is born to a healthy woman. A healthy woman evolves from a healthy girl and a healthy girl comes from a healthy community."

Dandelion Africa doesn't begin their work at pregnancy; they start by changing attitudes and healthcare options in their community. They focus on women's empowerment, school and youth leadership programs, and integrated health services.

Even with all of these services, six out of ten women in their neighborhood and surrounding area delivered their babies unattended at home. Dandelion Africa desperately needed a maternity ward to close the loop of women's healthcare for their community. This maternity ward became one of the projects of our No Mom Left Behind Campaign.

While we were visiting, one of our staff members, Theresa Greer, sat down with local women and asked if they wanted to share their own stories of childbirth. At the time the finishing touches were being done on the building and it officially opened to the community right after our visit. All of these stories were experienced before the new maternity ward opened.

Before it opened, women shared that they had to walk ten miles while in labor to get to the Mogotio Hospital. On arrival, they were often harassed or beaten by the doctors and left outside because they couldn't afford the fees.

Many women, like Margaret, didn't make it the ten miles; she ended up delivering her baby on the road, just trying to get to the hospital. Margaret had to ask a little boy who was walking by to help her cut the umbilical cord.

"You know," she said, "some are not so lucky. My friend's baby died being born on the road."

Another woman, Caroline, didn't even try to make it to the hospital; she delivered at home because she didn't want to risk the walk and couldn't afford the fees. Caroline delivered at home, unattended. She gave herself her own episiotomy, cut her own umbilical cord, and massaged her own stomach to stop the bleeding.

Not only is this excruciating and dangerous, it also does nothing to prevent mother-to-child transmission of HIV. With the knowledge we have today, no baby needs to be born HIV-positive. None. There are drugs available that reduce mother-to-child transmission to nearly zero. But these drugs need to be accessible, and assessing a mother's HIV status should be part of her prenatal care. This care needs to be available to all women—everywhere.

While we were visiting, we asked Wendo why she named their organization after the dandelion:

> When we were researching what to call the organization, we were looking for something that represents the resilience of women, our beauty, how we wear many hats.
>
> The dandelion plant is not only stubborn, it is resilient, medicinal, beautiful and everything women represent. We face adversity, but we always have the ability to blow and grow somewhere else. We grow in the most unlikely places. We are wonderfully made; one can use everything we have to offer, our hearts, our wit, our compassion, just like the dandelion—all its parts can be used. In Kenya, the dandelion is even used for blood cleaning; that is, if you have an infection, you are given the dandelion roots or tea to cleanse your system.

That is what this name stands for: what we are as women and what we as an organization believe in. I commonly say, it is not the thunder that grows flowers, but the rain. The dandelion is the rain, not the thunder; while we are disregarded as women, oppressed, abused, we are the rain that makes flowers grow.

I have never looked at a dandelion the same way again.

As we left the clinic, I noticed a sign on their wall that caught my attention. It said, *What are we here for, if not to help each other?* I have opened and closed whole speeches with that quote ever since I saw it. It's the truth.

The No Mom Left Behind Campaign was something that our team looked forward to every year. The idea of providing services and infrastructure specific to the needs of moms, building organizations that focused on newborns, children, and mothers, changed the future of entire communities.

A parent in Kenya or Uganda or India has the same love, the same aspirations, and the same dreams for their child that I have for my grandchild. That baby being born on the side of the road in Kenya right now is just as valuable as that baby being born right now at Swedish Hospital in Seattle, with a freaking Starbucks in the lobby.

30/30 PROJECT

CONCLUSIONS

If you change the way you look at things,
the things you look at change.

Wayne Dyer

During our second trip to Kenya, we had a couple of days to rest so we splurged and relaxed at a beautiful lakeside resort on Lake Victoria. The lake was gorgeous to look at, but unfortunately, not one we could swim in, nor could we sink our feet into the sandy beach. As lovely as Lake Victoria is, the shore is full of parasitic worms that our Western immune system, especially mine, can't handle. The water in Lake Victoria, though vital to the livelihood of about thirty million people in East Africa, has increasing pollution levels, and some parts are covered with a green carpet composed of propagated water hyacinths. Needless to say, the water was also something that I couldn't be exposed to.

While at the resort, Laura and I stayed in a beautiful thatched hut with a cone-shaped ceiling. Inside, our beds were surrounded by a zippered square enclosure made of mosquito netting. We noticed when putting our stuff away that there were more than a few cute little geckos wandering around, inside and out. In the middle of the first night, we began to hear popping sounds on the roof of our sleeping tent, a bit of a splatter sound.

Through the dimly moonlit room, Laura asked me, "Do you hear that weird sound?"

"Yes." I listened as the plopping sound continued. "It is strange. What do you think it is?"

Laura was silent for a moment, as if thinking and taking in all the possibilities. Then she replied with a creepy factor in her voice, "Gecko poop. I think the geckos are pooping above us."

She was right. Gecko poop was raining down, falling from the high ceilings and landing with a "plop" on the top of our mosquito net enclosure. The next day we adjusted, closing our suitcases and laying towels on top of our laptops at night.

Staying at that resort was a true reminder that as privileged Westerners, we live such clean and sanitized lives, in more ways than one. I've come to think that this luxury of ease and plenty has left us somewhat weak. I saw real strength and hardiness, wisdom and fortitude in the beautiful people I met in Kenya. Our reality of living sterile lives in the US is not always a blessing when it leads to a sense of entitlement and greed.

I confess that when I saw the word "resort," I had expectations. Those expectations did not include parasitic worms and gecko poop. I began to see very clearly that I had relatively little stamina in the face of everyday inconveniences. As I write this, in the middle of the coronavirus pandemic, I am seeing the disservice we've created for ourselves here in the US, being used to getting everything we need instantly and, if not, complaining until things go the way we wish.

During the five years of the 30/30 Project, we did experience setbacks. I'm making sure to include this because

I believe that we often don't do things because we're afraid of failure, afraid that not everything will go well. We're also fearful that if we share what went wrong, that it takes away from everything that went right. I think sharing our setbacks and what we learned from them is healthy and good. Hopefully it encourages others to name what hasn't worked in their lives and jobs, to learn from those disappointments, and to move on. One of our healthcare clinics that we built early on in the project did not open for almost five years. There were many reasons for this, including us needing to improve our initial vetting process. The good news is that we continued to communicate with this community, and today the clinic is providing vital services.

Recently, in Seattle, I saw a woman wearing red shoes and baggy sweatpants courageously walking sideways across a five-way intersection to make her journey the shortest possible, despite what the traffic lights and crosswalk signs were suggesting. She had a limp and seemed to be struggling to just cross on the shortest route. As I watched her, I had great admiration and waited my turn, not according to the traffic signals; I waited for something much more valuable, this woman's well-being.

The whole scene, as it unfolded, reminded me of many groups we had the privilege to work with throughout the 30/30 Project. Sometimes, immediately upon dedicating a healthcare building in a community, we were asked, at that very dedication ceremony, for more money. We were often pitched a new idea or plan and asked for funding for additional buildings to be built. Some people would take that as our partner organizations and partner communities being ungrateful. I have grown to admire the effort and gutsiness to ask immediately, using the shortest route possible to get what that organization and community need. Most of these health facilities are in areas around the world where future options for growth are few. I've come to see these requests, not as being rude or ungrateful, but as a strength. Just like the woman in the intersection, these organizations get my attention and respect when they know their needs and solutions.

In fact, our whole 30/30 team noticed when organizations were not passive, or even at times polite, in an effort to move their goals forward. We had greater confidence that they would go to great effort to maintain their buildings and sustain their work. Those organizations had a lot of grit and pluck because they didn't always follow the rules to the letter.

Here's the thing that our partners understood about healthcare: Even though this was called the 30/30 Project, these were not just "projects" to them. To many of our partners, these healthcare buildings were about life or death. Bringing health to their communities was so much more than bringing buildings and providing medicine. To our partners, these buildings represented options and access for everyone. They represented equity and equality. Quality of life and quantity of life. They represented power. Decision-making power. Education. Gaining the knowledge and facts to make the best decisions for themselves and their families. They were also about creating opportunity, a chance for community members to live productive lives.

Sometimes in life, every piece of one's past and all of the parts of one's present manage to fit together in a way that makes the outcome much more than the mere sum of its parts. The 30/30 Project brought together my illness and experience being a woman infected with HIV, my experience teaching, my quest as a health educator, and my passion for public health. It added in Scott's and my lifetime of experience working for and with nonprofits, our moving to Seattle at a time when Ryan could focus on his art and music, Jenny and me volunteering for Construction for Change, which taught us about infrastructure needs around the world. It wove together Ryan's hard work, timing, fame, and good fortune in performing on a world stage, the platform he gained having a successful album and career, and access not only to his fans, but also to the media. All of these pieces together allowed the 30/30 Project to not just succeed but to thrive.

At the end of five years, together with Construction for Change, the 30/30 Project partnered to build thirty healthcare facilities for eighteen different organizations in nine countries, including the US and Puerto Rico.

Hopefully, in building these health centers, we have created a ripple of hope, a ripple of justice, and a ripple of equality.

I believe that there isn't such a thing as someone else's child or someone else's mother. That child in Malawi or India is our child. That mom, whether in Kenya or on the streets of Seattle, is our mother. We are all in this world together.

What are we here for if not to help each other?

TRADITIONS 2.0

It's a delight
when all your imaginations come true.

L.M. Montgomery, Anne of Green Gables

That first year in the '90s when we decided to sit on pillows around the coffee table with three small kids for Christmas Eve salmon dinner, I never expected to be enjoying the same tradition so many years later. The coffee table has become more and more crowded as our family grew; we were joined by boyfriends, girlfriends, and finally the spouses of all three of our grown children. As much as I try, no one wants to give up our silly tradition for the comfort of the dining room table. Some traditions you pick; some you're stuck with.

Everyone in our family would agree that Christmas would not be the same without sharing our highs and lows. We've had some low lows, as we lost friends and family members over the years. But back when we started the tradition, I never dreamed that one day I would still be here for the Christmas Eve when Teresa announced that her "high for the year" was that moment and getting to tell Scott and me that we would become grandparents for the first time!

Now, I have six grandchildren whom we've introduced to the tradition of Christmas highs and lows and for whom I now buy special ornaments and PJs for every Christmas. Even though we've had to occasionally switch dates, or, this past year, manage with part of the family joining via Zoom, we've kept the tradition.

Last year, at our family Christmas celebration, Teresa handed out presents to Ryan, Laura, Scott, and me. We all opened them at the same time; there in front of each of us was a beautiful watercolor print of the fountain at Duncan Gardens where Scott had told them I had HIV. That was over twenty-five years ago but it had been the beginning of their AIDS journey, and now each of us had a beautiful image to hang on the wall to remember. We all got a little teary-eyed looking at that fountain and realizing just how much we had survived, but even more so, how grateful we were to still be together.

Collectively, we looked forward to these times every year; we cherished them and guarded them. In the world of AIDS, where all of us were constantly aware that life could take so much, we built something that couldn't be stolen from us: special memories.

DR. DEBBIE

The meaning of life is to find your gift.
The purpose of life is to give it away.

Picasso

When I turned sixty, my family made me a very special scrapbook with notes from my friends and family. I was touched by the kind words people sent my way as I started my next decade.

The most profound note was not the longest; in fact, it was fairly short. It was from my friend Debbie:

> Julie,
>
> I have a bond with you on many levels like no one else. My life direction changed the day we became friends.
>
> I love you,
>
> Debbie

When I moved to Seattle from Spokane, the person I missed most was definitely Debbie. But, being part of my extended family, I knew I would see her and that we were bonded for life. In our ten years of living in the same neighborhood and working in the same community, she had been my daily comrade. She was there in the effort to prevent and educate regarding the spread of HIV and also in my personal and spiritual life as a mom and spouse.

When Debbie moved to Spokane in 1994, she was a dietician, and by the time I moved to Seattle, she had become the Adherence Treatment Coordinator at the Spokane AIDS Network.

The really remarkable thing happened after I moved, when Debbie started down the path of becoming a physician's assistant. I was so impressed. We were not exactly young people, and she was going back to school and changing her career in a major way. Not only did she become a PA, but Debbie became a specialist in HIV treatment.

Since becoming a physician's assistant, she has dedicated the last fifteen years working as a key HIV provider in the greater Spokane area. Debbie partnered with the University of Washington Medical Center to provide the highest quality of care available to her HIV-infected patients.

There have been very few people, other than Scott and the kids, who have been there from the start to the end of this story. Many people have come in and out of my life over the years and some, like my brother Chris, are part of my blood and can't ever be divorced from my life. But, the one person who has been part of so many of my stories, from HIV to advocacy, from raising kids to my dad dying, has been Debbie.

To have such a good friend and relative right down the street in those scariest days of AIDS was something I never knew I needed, something I didn't plan. Looking back, that relationship changed everything for the better.

TRUTH VS. FICTION

Love one another.

John 13:24

In 1993, I decided to write a series of essays for my kids, stories they could read about me after I died. I didn't anticipate that I would survive longer than expected; by the time I began public speaking with the speakers' bureau, I ended up putting those notes for my kids away in a drawer.

Several years ago, I gave those essays to Teresa to read.

When she was done, she asked, "Who is this woman?"

What I hadn't anticipated was that no matter how much I wanted to write something to my two-year-old, four-year-old, or six-year-old that they might read as their adult self, it was very hard to imagine that small child as an adult; and that skewed my writing. I think what Teresa was reading, what I wrote when I was her age, as a young, dying mom of small kids, showed someone who was starkly different from the "fuck this" mom she's used to.

The mom Teresa is accustomed to is honest, opinionated, political, and sometimes overly analytical. I'm not insinuating that I'm not nice or that I try to behave inappropriately. I just don't spend a great deal of effort sugarcoating things like I did in those stories, when I was writing to my two-year-old.

I decided to read through those stories after Teresa did. As I was reading, I began to see, pretty clearly, that most of the essays, topics, and stories were really a huge document of bargaining with God.

Everything, and I mean every story and problem, was solved by a Bible verse and a faith message. It was incredible how I spun every topic to have a positive God ending. Nothing could end sadly; it was all going to work for God's good, and I would find every silver lining possible. It was a bit of a *Chicken Soup for the Soul: Personal Dying Edition.*

I was begging, trying to strike a deal with God, saying, "If I spin everything in my life to have great faith, maybe God will let me live longer."

I threw that book in the trash several years ago, right after Teresa's analysis. I was a little embarrassed and feared that someone might get a hold of it and judge me accordingly. When I began to write this story, I regretted not having those thoughts written right in the thick of the beginning years of living with HIV.

Then last January, almost thirty years after I wrote it, Teresa's special person, Gloria, said, "Oh I have a copy of what you wrote for your kids in the bottom drawer of my desk. I'll make sure to send it to you."

I couldn't believe she'd saved it.

When I think back to the early 1990s when I wrote those notes, I just wanted to have it all figured out. I wanted to read the books on grief and loss and get over it. Maybe not over it but beyond it. I wanted to have answers to complicated questions. Unanswerable things. I wanted to wrap it in a package, tie a bow, and say this is what I've learned. This is what God is doing. This is why everything happened.

Here I am years later, and I can confidently say that just doesn't happen. That's not real. None of us can know or understand everything. There is no way to figure it all out. I can't write a book that's going to tell people what to do or how to manage a medical or family crisis. I feel like the more life experience I have, the less "how to do it" kind of dialogue I really believe in.

The advantage to a fictional story is that there is control over everything. It can all be made palatable and, in some way, take the reader to the edge without sending them over the cliff. Everything in fiction can be tied up. Real life, on the other hand, has too many layers; so many things that are left hanging. It's messy.

In my own story, there are many things in thirty years that are unresolved and seem unresolvable—why did a blood transfusion intended to save my life completely rewrite it; why did Chris and I live when so many others died; why would God allow a seven-year-old to die instead of someone like me; why was I not explained the risks of a blood transfusion in 1984 and given a choice as to whether I wanted to take that risk; should we have waited longer to tell the kids; how could we have parented differently to lessen the stress and worry on our children? This list could keep going; the questions are unending.

This book may be my final effort to let those complicated, real-life stories and reflections rest on the page and find some kind of finality, a peaceful spot from which I can move on. Perhaps these stories can propel survivors forward toward the beautiful, messed up world we all call home and away from dwelling on the past.

Perhaps we can find peace and joy in the imperfection of life in general, to find grace and forgiveness, to hold things lightly and people tightly. To admit that we are human, we are flawed, and we are destined for and capable of love and great works. To dare to believe that God even cares. That God, in fact, not only created this human condition, but even loves and enjoys us, despite the chaos.

This brings me to the core of why I believe in God. Sometimes, in life, we are trapped in our own understanding of who we think we are. How we perceive the world seems to come out of that self-analysis. I, myself, am critical and scrutinize my life often, focusing on what needs to change. The thing is, change is hard; I don't get very far trying to change anything on my own.

The biggest reason I believe in God is that when I stop and just give up, God seems to meet me in that space and lets me know it's okay, I'm okay. I am softened in that space and reminded to forgive myself. We are all flawed, but the good news is that God loves flawed people.

Without God, everything seems hollow to me. I don't want to be hollow or live a hollow life. God chooses to love us despite ourselves. God lives at our core and then also all around us and beyond all we can imagine. Deep inside there is a compulsion, a drawing me in toward the bigger, deeper mystery, to a reality where I am both incredibly small and insignificant while at the same time precious and valued. When I look to the mountains and to the night sky, I sense that God is immense, and yet when I ponder that each snowflake is individually distinct, I see that God cares about details. That this God would choose to include me in those details, care about my life, and want to commune with me is kind of crazy, and yet here I am, skeptic of skeptics, believing this to be true. I need God like I need air, water, food.

To me, God is love. God can display love often through people and circumstances. God's love sometimes comes from the most unlikely sources, it doesn't have conditions, and it can feel like soothing ointment on a gaping wound. If we are lucky, God uses us to spread love to others.

In one form or another, I've been a Christian my whole life. Lutheran growing up, then diving headfirst into evangelical Christianity in college and staying there, both through church and through our involvement with youth ministry on and off for a large part of my life.

All the while, I've been bouncing back and forth into the constraints of this version of Christian culture. Rubbing up on the edges where my version of faith and God didn't fit into the box laid out before me. After Scott and I were married, even before AIDS zapped the energy out of me, I struggled to fit into the role of "supportive wife" that was expected of me. And then I became the AIDS lady, preaching safe sex in schools and attending a church on the weekend that was preaching abstinence.

Looking back, the reason Scott, Debbie, and I felt the need to start a "Christian" support group was because I wanted the Georges and Barrys and all of the others who had been hurt by churches to know that there were Christians out there who loved them and accepted them for who they were. That God would create HIV as a punishment for being gay is unfathomable and heretical—no matter how many misguided people preached it from pulpits around the world. I wanted them to know that.

I knew that the church could sometimes be slow to catch up to culture, or more clearly, human rights. I was waiting for it. Forty years later, I'm still waiting for much of the church to catch up. Even today, several of the Christian organizations that Scott and I worked for and volunteered with still are not inclusive and supportive of LGBTQ+ people and have hurtful, discriminatory policies around leadership and employment. Some churches still refuse to ordain women and consider them second class to men. I've watched divorced white men lead large Christian organizations while writing policies that shame and isolate. They weaponize Bible verses when judging others but use a scale of grace when judging themselves.

It's no longer acceptable for me to stay within the confines of those organizations who claim to "love everyone" yet watch them actively turn away those who are not like them, who don't fit into their box. I dare to believe that God created each of us exactly as we are, and God's love is not discriminatory nor exclusionary just because God's children don't check certain boxes.

A while back, I had a taste of the love of God and what it might mean when the Bible says, "become like little children."

On that day, one of my grandsons got locked inside his family car with the keys, too young to figure out how to unlock the door himself. When he was telling me the story later, he said, "My dad got locked out of the car."

I thought about that for a while. Almost any adult would have said, "I got locked inside the car."

But not Mylo. For him, it wasn't his problem, it was his dad's. He wasn't scared at all because he trusted that his dad, who locked himself out of the car, would figure out how to get back inside the car and get him out.

I think this is a beautiful analogy to faith and the love God has for each of us. Even though life is difficult, and we often feel "stuck" inside the car, God loves all of us, as our eternal parent, and God will always find a way to reach us. I'm trying to trust this God of love to get us out of the car. To bring us safely beyond our many obstacles, beyond the things that knock us down, beyond life that is out of our control, beyond ourselves—one way or another.

MOM

There are only two lasting bequests
we can hope to give our children.
One of these is roots, the other, wings.

Johann Wolfgang von Goethe

My mom died in December of 2019. She'd been living in a long-term care facility for five years dealing with Alzheimer's, such a baffling disease, erasing bits and fragments of memory but not in a predictable or logical way. In the end my mom couldn't remember my name, but somehow, she could put together a five-hundred-piece jigsaw puzzle with her friend Ed. I would find her sleeping later, clutching some of the puzzle pieces in her hand. They felt like a representation of the parts of herself that she seemed desperate to hold on to.

Right before Christmas, she fell and broke her hip; four days later she was gone. Her last "meal" was a taste of a York peppermint patty, and her last request to the chaplain was prayer for "protection." When going through her things I found more of those lost puzzle orphans in her bed linens, tiny jigsaw pieces that would never be reunited with the bigger picture. I took a few of them home and put them inside a heart box sitting on my desk.

I've been thinking about Mom often, everything from reminiscing about my days with her as a kid, her last-born child, to wondering what she was asking for exactly when she wanted prayer for "protection" before she died. Was she wanting protection for herself or for those of us left behind? Some things I'll never know; some questions die when the only person who can answer them is gone.

My mom's fortitude was remarkable. After my dad passed in 2002, my mom spent seventeen years living alone, most of those years in a remote and isolated place. It had to be so lonely. She had to be fearful. How did she do it? What did she do with all of her time? I know she spent hours reading; she kept a typed list of well over two hundred books she'd finished. But still, she had no FaceTime, no social media, no Netflix. My mom and I were never super close, but the older I get, I find myself facing fears of isolation and loneliness; I admire her resilience and regret that I wasn't more present in her life those last few years.

Thinking back to the day we told my parents that Chris and I were expecting to die from AIDS, I knew it would be devastating news for them. At least, I thought I knew. Now that I'm the same age that my parents were then and have kids who are the same age that we were when we told them, I see that I really had no idea how devastating this must have been for my parents. Relating it to my life now, if Ryan were to show up at our house today and tell Scott and me that both he and Laura had a disease that they were going to die from in the next couple years, I would be beyond devastated.

But on that day, the day we dropped the kids off in Yakima and went to tell my parents, I was so into my own personal life and my concern for our kids, I really didn't think of how a sixty-year-old would take this news about their thirty-something-year-old kids.

Later, when my dad and I were reflecting back on that day, he said to me, "It doesn't matter if your kids are five years old or thirty-five, the worst thing in life is to lose your kids."

I get that now.

My mom never was able to talk much about Chris's and my diagnoses even though she was the one who first suggested the possibility that I was infected with HIV. I guess when the idea turned into reality, it became too hard for her to say out loud, like her silence could somehow make it go away. I never held that against her. Sometimes in life, denial is an appropriate response.

As I was writing this chapter, I paused to look out my bedroom window, and a deer came down the hill outside and walked straight toward me, staring at me. It got so close to my window. For a split second I had the thought that the deer was my mom checking on me, letting me know she was fine and making sure I was okay. I smiled and waved and blew a kiss. Then she walked slowly away, looking back a couple of times. I'm not a believer in reincarnation, but I do have faith in signs and imagery. I will never forget that encounter.

I am so grateful that my parents' worst nightmare never materialized. They didn't live to watch any of their children die. I hope and pray I'm as fortunate.

WHO TELLS YOUR STORY

The universe is made of stories, not of atoms.

Muriel Rukeyser

Everything can change in an instant. In the first week of March 2020, trying to avoid Seattle, which had become the US epicenter of a new pandemic, I moved from my house to Ryan's cabin in a remote area of Central Washington. I wrote much of this book during those early days of COVID-19.

Watching the pandemic unfold and our sense of "normal" changing daily, reminded me of my early days of HIV. In reliving my HIV diagnosis, at first there was the reeling from all of the worst-case possibilities and the unknown. And then came despair that life was forever changed, a realization that I am, in fact, not invincible. That awareness was accompanied by strict protocols to relieve fear and keep people around me as healthy as possible. The beginnings of COVID-19 felt eerily similar.

The pandemic has made me profoundly aware that upending change has been happening throughout the ages, be it disease, or war, or natural disasters; people are displaced around the world all the time. It's just I hadn't experienced anything so disruptive on such a massive global scale. I'm sure I am not alone; many of us have gotten a taste of what much of our world has been born into for generations. We've seen our broken systems exposed and highlighted in the midst of a new level of need and disaster.

Although the isolation of the remote cabin created challenging circumstances to try to live a productive life, it also made me aware that not everyone could escape to such a vacuum. I became lonely; nonetheless, I also realized that I am incredibly privileged. One of the things I did every day during my isolation was to take long walks down a winding dirt road, meandering through several pear orchards. I kept Ryan's Doberman, Scarlett, at my side after several cougars had been spotted in the canyon.

Audiobooks kept me company, my favorite being *Anne Frank: The Diary of a Young Girl,* read by Selma Blair. So, when I felt sorry for myself, for my own solitary existence, missing my husband, kids, and grandkids, I listened to Anne who, as a Jewish teenager during WWII, spent almost two years in an attic with seven other people, hoping to stay alive. Anne Frank was an incredible writer, brutally honest in the best way.

I fell in love with Anne Frank. I loved that she spent a whole chapter on what she would buy if she could go to a department store with unlimited resources. I love that she figured out how to be creative with her time, how she found humor in most things and yet didn't minimize the horror of what was happening every day around her.

Anne reminded me that we don't need much: food, shelter, health, and relationships. There's so much wasted time, money, and energy on stuff, on things. In the middle of my isolation, all I wanted was to hug my kids and grandkids again, share a meal, and know that we were all safe. I'm pretty sure that's what everyone wants, everywhere.

Then I remembered my weird little bunny pen that I randomly grew fond of writing with, and I thought about the blue jay who often sat on the split-wood fence in the yard, and I'm mindful that sometimes it's the little things that give us joy and remind us that there's something to appreciate, to love, to look forward to. Anne's diary pointed out constantly that small things matter.

Maybe it's the collection of small things that enable us to get through and do the bigger, harder things that life serves up.

As I listened to Anne Frank, and as I read daily stories of loss from the pandemic, I saw many feelings, thoughts, and actions that have crossed over from one challenging era to the next. I saw inspiration that wasn't frozen in time—it reached across generations, shedding hope, and providing comfort. Anne was my ally, my encouragement, and through my listening to her story, in a small sense, I was hers.

Anne Frank wrote in her diary, "I wish someday I could write something great." At the time she was writing a classic. *The Diary of Anne Frank* has sold over thirty million copies and has been translated into seventy different languages.

I don't think we see our moments of greatness when we are in the middle of them. Maybe we are all having our "moment" right now. Maybe this day will contain our "something great," and we just can't see it. Anne Frank did not live to see her great moment as a writer, but she did get to tell her own story.

Her story was her greatness.

What stands out to me in hard times are the stories. The stories of real people living real lives. I am reminded of the verse from the musical *Hamilton*, where George Washington says, "You have no control, who lives, who dies, who tells your story."

Living with AIDS in the 1990s was a lot like that. There was no real way to predict who would live, who would die, and who would tell your story. A few of us survived by taking a boatload of medicine and by being lucky. Too many were not so lucky: Joyce, Kara, Camie, Mary, George, Barry, Mark, Craig, Harold, and countless others, did not make it.

This book and the 30/30 Project are dedicated to these friends in an effort to remember them, to honor them, and to continue to tell their stories.

My life's journey constantly leaves me with more questions than answers, but I do know this: I love God, I love people, and God loves all of us—every single one of us.

My family, my friends, and my community are what have made my life great. They've given me beauty and purpose and have filled my days with meaning and love.

That's my story.

ACKNOWLEDGMENTS

Ryan was the one who first encouraged me to write my memoir. It was the fall of 2019, and the funds for all thirty of our 30/30 Project healthcare facilities had been raised, so I asked him what he thought I should do next. "Write the book", he said. So that fall, having no book writing experience, I started drawing up an outline.

Little did I know that COVID was about to hit. I'm not going to lie, I was very unsure I would survive COVID at first, and wanting to at least get the story down in its roughest form and knowing someone else could fix it later, my writing went into hyper speed and I finished the first edition in May of 2020.

That was a long time ago, and the book has been worked and reworked, edited, and re-edited many times since. I probably would not have kept going, at times being so frustrated, but in early 2021 Jenny Koenig stepped in to be my writing partner, and this book project went from feeling impossible to being a fun adventure. Thank you, Jenny, you are a true gift to me and such a talented writer. I look forward to the books, movie scripts, and screenplays you will bestow upon us in the future.

Jenny and I want to thank the team at Light Messages and Torchflame Books, especially our editor Elizabeth Turnbull. As first-time book writers, Jenny and I have learned so much as you have walked us through the book publishing process.

We have felt patience, grace, and expertise bestowed on us by our publishing family. We truly won the book writers' lottery by being chosen as one of your 2023 publications.

Ian Goode, you hit the ball out of the park with the book cover design! Thank you for the creativity, time, and love you put into our original vision, it exceeded all our expectations.

Thank you also to the many people who read our manuscript along the way, giving us encouragement and vitally needed suggestions and edits. Kristine, Kelly, Ed (and the other Ed), Dave and Teresa, Kathy, Danielle, Teresa G, Jim and Patty, Christina, Ashley, Chris, Alex, Barbara, Kelsey, and Debbie. You kept us on task and continually let us know that what we were writing mattered.

When I began to write about the speakers' bureau, I knew it was going to draw up many memories and feelings, not only for myself but also for the community that supported each other through an extreme period of loss. In the book, I wanted to capture the true voices of my friends who had passed as accurately as possible. What an unexpected surprise to find that my coworker, Julie Zink, had saved word-for-word manuscripts of speeches we all had given in the early 1990s, almost every newspaper clipping that featured a speaker, and videotapes of speaking events. Thank you, Julie, for just handing those over to me with your blessing. You have been a true advocate like none other, and I treasure our thirty years of friendship.

I also want to thank the surviving family members who have let me share their loved one's experiences, some memories carrying with them sadness and pain. I hope I have honored their lives by showing the brave way they shared their stories in an effort to educate people during an age of fear and discrimination. They are my heroes.

I'm not sure what I thought parenting adult children and being a grandmother would be like in my younger years, but it is far more incredible than I could ever have imagined. My kids; Teresa, Laura, and Ryan, have become my loyal cheerleaders, my most honest mentors, my biggest supporters, and my closest friends. Over the last ten years, both through the 30/30 Project and while Jenny and I wrote this book, they have each helped in different ways by reading, editing, helping with social media, and leading creative content, including the book cover design. I am such a lucky mom to be able to observe and sometimes be included in each of my kids' individual places of influence. I love their families, and it is pure joy when we have time together. Thank you does not seem big enough to express my love and appreciation for all three of you, your spouses (Patrick, Alex, and Jackie), and our crew of grandkids... Mylo, Rory, Fiona, Luna, Ramona, and Ruby... I just want to say that I love you all from the bottom of my heart.

I am ending my thanks with the person who has been my anchor and rock for over forty years now. Scott; my partner in all things, love of my life, true companion, loyal friend, lifter of my spirit, encourager like no other, best father ever, the person who cries with me, laughs out loud in the middle of the night, calms my fears, knows my secrets and always supports my crazy ideas. He took those vows seriously, the "in sickness and in health" part, and has been with me on this journey in ways I can never fully explain in a book. The biggest thing I did right in life was to say yes to sharing our lives together, something I thank God for every day. I love you, and I know that you will always be there with that "extended hug"... and be the one who forever has my back.

My life has been full of God's blessings and showered with God's mercy... I have been fortunate to receive an abundance of both. I thank God for this gift of life, and I hope to never take it for granted, never take myself too seriously, and always create space to see the miracles that happen every day.

JULIE LEWIS

Julie is a 39-year AIDS survivor, and mother to Grammy Award-winning music producer, Ryan Lewis. She was infected with HIV in 1984 but not diagnosed until the early 1990s, when she was given three to five years to live. After years of silence about her disease, she found an unlikely community of friends to fight alongside and 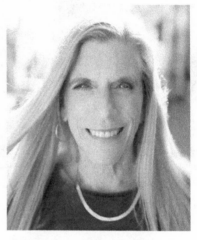 began using her story to make a difference. Her experiences as a woman living with AIDS offer insights about grief and loss, caregiving, spirituality, and the importance of community in the midst of tragedy.

Thirty years later, wanting to find a way to celebrate her incredible journey, and her passion for community health, she launched the 30/30 Project to positively impact the lives of other women, girls, and families who didn't have the same access to the healthcare opportunities that she's had.

The five-year project has resulted in 30 healthcare facilities, built for 18 organizations in 9 countries, including the US and Puerto Rico.

Julie has shared her story on CBS This Morning, Anderson Cooper, and The Elvis Duran Show. Julie, a recipient of the Nelson Mandela Change-maker Award, has opened international conferences and has been the keynote speaker at several events focused on healthcare, empowering women, and uplifting communities whose voices need to be amplified.

JENNY KOENIG

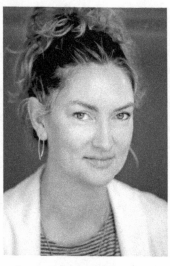

Jenny is a writer and Grammy Nominated Music Video Producer. She's passionate about channeling her creativity into ways to raise money for nonprofits, including the 30/30 Project. She was a co-creator and Executive Producer for All in WA: A Concert for COVID Relief, which raised over $110 million for COVID-related causes. She's learning how to juggle life as a new mom to her 6-month-old daughter. Jenny is a longtime friend of Julie Lewis and jumped at the chance to help her tell her story.

Proceeds from *Still Positive* are donated to organizations focusing on healthcare access, issues, and equity.

Follow Julie and Jenny
https://stillpositive.com
Instagram @stillpositivebook

SOURCES REFERENCED

THE QUESTION OF BLAME

Leveton LB, Sox HC Jr. and Stoto MA. "HIV and the Blood Supply: An Analysis of Crisis Decision Making." *Institute of Medicine (US) Committee to Study HIV Transmission Through Blood and Blood Products.* 1995 ncbi.nlm.nih.gov/books/ NBK232419/. sections 3,4,5.

McGraw, Carol. "Some AIDS Victims Win Blood Cases." *L.A. Times*, 16 Sept. 1990. https://www.latimes.com/archives/la-xpm-1990-09-16-mn-1224-story.html.

Talaverna, Jessamine R.."Quintana v. United Blood Services: Examining Industry and Practice in Transfusion Related AIDS Cases. *Cornell Journal of Law and Public Policy*, Vol. 2, Issue 2, Article 7. Spring 1993. https://scholarship.law.cornell.edu/cgi/ viewcontent.cgi?article=1152&context=cjlpp.

JOYCE

Johnson, Carla K. "Experts say secrecy is no solution." Spokesman Review, August 29, 1993, p. A11.

Johnson, Carla K. "Mom fights fear with honesty." Spokesman Review, August 29, 1993, p. A1.

SUPPORT GROUP

Pate, Suzanne. "In a Huff." POZ Magazine, October 1, 1997.

CAMIE AND WORLD AIDS DAY

Endo, Emi. "HIV-Infected Women Make Plea For AIDS Education." Spokesman Review, February 18, 1995.

A HAMBURGER

Durvasula, Ramani and Kelly Ebeling. "A History of HIV/ AIDS in Women: Shifting Narrative and a Structural Call to Arms." *Psychology and AIDS Exchange Newsletter*, Mar. 2018. https://www.apa.org/pi/aids/resources/exchange/2018/03/ history-women.

Wilder, Terri. "A Timeline of Women Living With HIV: Past, Present and Future." *The Body: The HIV/AIDS Resource*, 13 May 2012. https://www.thebody.com/article/a-timeline-of- women-living-with-hiv-past-present-a-23.

"Impact of the Expanded AIS Surveillance Case Definition on AIDS Case Reporting -- United States, First Quarter, 1993." *CDC, MMWR Weekly*, 30 Apr. 1993. https://www.cdc.gov/ mmwr/preview/mmwrhtml/00020374.htm.

ACTUP https://en.wikipedia.org/wiki/ACT_UP . Accessed 1 Sept 2021.

COLORADO SPRINGS

Bailey Boushay House https://en.wikipedia.org/wiki/Bailey- Boushay_House

Colorado Amendment 2 https://coloradoencyclopedia.org/ article/amendment-2

KARA

Johnson, Carla K. "A Year Of Joy, Tears, Despite Battle With AIDS, Kara Claypool Moves Ahead." Spokesman Review, June 19, 1995

Johnson, Carla K. "Spokane Loses littlest Hero Kara Claypool Dies Of Disease She Helped Us Accept." Spokesman Review, August 31, 1995, p. A1.

NEW YORK

Broadway CARES https://broadwaycares.org/broadway- cares-awards-record-breaking-grants-despite-pandemic- setbacks

THE QUILT

Dunlap, David W. "AIDS Quilt of Grief on Capital Mall." New York Times, 13 Oct. 1996. https://www.nytimes.com/1996/10/13/us/aids-quilt-of-grief-on-capital-mall.html.

The NAMES Project https://en.wikipedia.org/wiki/NAMES_Project_AIDS_Memorial_Quilt

THE DAWN OF A NEW ERA

Hyatt, Michael S. Y2K: What Every Christian Should Know. (Nelson Audio Library, April 1, 1999).

DISCLOSURE

Americans with Disabilities ACT https://archive.ada.gov/hiv/index.html

SACRED CIRCUMSTANCES AND TRIVIAL COINCIDENCES

The NIV Study Bible, 10th Anniversary Edition. (The Zondervan Corporation, 1995.) 716

DEPRESSION AND COPING

Makkai, Rebecca. The Great Believers. (Viking, First Edition, 19 June 2018) 260, 253.

COLLATERAL DAMAGE

Johnson, Emma and Margaret DeMonte. "One Family's Secret: Our Parents Died of AIDS." Glamour Magazine, 31 Oct. 2006. https://www.glamour.com/story/parents-living-with-aids.

THE 30/30 PROJECT

Kidder, Tracy. Mountains Beyond Mountains, The Quest Of Dr. Paul Farmer, A Man Who Would Cure The World. (Random House, 2003).

MANDELAS

Mandela, Ndaba. Going to the Mountain: Life Lessons from My Grandfather, Nelson Mandela. (Hachette Books, 26 Jun 2018) 207.

NO MOM LEFT BEHIND

Tikkanen R, Gunja MZ, FitzGerald M and Zephyrin L. "Maternal Mortality and Maternal Care in the United States Compared to 10 Other Developed Countries." The Commonwealth Fund, 18 Nov. 2020. https://www.commonwealthfund.org/publications/issue-briefs/2020/nov/maternal-mortality-maternity-care-us-compared-10-countries.

Fernandez, Maria Elena. "Why Black women are less likely to survive pregnancy, and what's being done about it." American Heart Association News, 10 Feb.2021. https://www.heart.org/en/news/2021/02/10/why-black-women-are-less-likely-to-survive-pregnancy-and-whats-being-done-about-it.

WHO TELLS YOUR STORY

Frank, Anne. Anne Frank: The Diary of a Young Girl: The Definitive Edition, narrated by Selma Blair. (Fingerprint Publishing, first edition June 25, 1947; Books on Tape Edition, May 25, 2010).

CPSIA information can be obtained
at www.ICGtesting.com
Printed in the USA
SHW081020020423
736JS00003B/15